Fear of Falling Phenomenology Study

Carol J. Bostic

ABSTRACT

Fear of falling (FoF) has been extensively studied in aging populations, due to the high prevalence of both falling and FoF in older adults. Research has identified a number of biological, psychological, and social/environmental factors related to the development of FoF. Research has yet to explore how FoF impacts the daily lives of caregiver and care recipient dyads along biological, psychological, and social/environmental domains. Existing literature also fails to provide clinicians, and in particular physical therapists, with considerations for the evaluation and clinical interviewing process for individuals seeking care related to FoF. This dissertation study is a phenomenology in which the essence of FoF was explored to understand the lived experiences of caregivers and care recipients who experience FoF within the dyadic relationship. Semi-structured interviews were conducted with four caregiver - care recipient dyads where at least one member of the dyad self-reported having FoF. An a priori code list, informed by the biopsychosocial model, was combined with an open analysis that assisted the principal investigator in gaining a deeper understanding of how FoF impacts the daily lives of older adults and their caregivers. Care recipient experiences with regard to FoF included: threats to autonomy, acceptance, maintenance of independence, and influence of the caregiver. Caregiver experiences with respect to caregiver concern for the care recipient falling included: burden of caregiving with respect to caregiver fall concern, compartmentalization during a fall emergency, , and reasons for caregiver fall concern. Lastly the experiences of the dyads were highlighted by the following themes: planning for the future and limiting burden. Communication regarding fall concerns, perception of care recipient fall risk and physical limitations were identified as potential sources of turbulence within the caregiving dyad. The results of this investigation suggest that the shared essence of FoF amongst study participants was the need to preserve their way of life. This investigation identified suggestions for the initial examination of individuals seeking physical therapy care regarding FoF and supports interdisciplinary treatment.

Keywords: Older adults, caregivers, fear of falling, biopsychosocial model, phenomenology

This work is dedicated to my family, study participants, patients, and to the 65+ community for inspiring me to do this work and become a better educator and clinician.

Acknowledgements

I would like to first and foremost begin by thanking my committee members, I would not have been able to complete this work without their guidance and commitment. Their timely feedback and constructive advice have allowed me to achieve the goals I have set for myself in this program. To Dr. Sarah Young, my chair: thank you for your unyielding commitment to my timeline of completion, and for directing me throughout this experience and for allowing me to grow in my confidence of using qualitative methodology through your guidance and teachings. Thank you for being open and willing to hear my ideas and allow me the opportunity to advocate for what I wanted to accomplish throughout this process. I cannot thank you enough for your willingness to serve in this role for me, and have no doubt that you will continue to guide doctoral students through the dissertation process. I would also like to thank Dr. Jackie McGinley for her guidance in giving me the tools to learn about caregiving literature, and for your 5am writing group to help me prepare to complete this work. I cannot thank you enough for our regular meetings and your kindness and support of me throughout this process. I wish to thank Dr. Youjung Lee for her guidance throughout the process and for helping me avoid pitfalls in conducting research with older adults. Finally, I would like to thank Dr. Michael Buck for stepping in to serve as my outside examiner. In addition, Mike, thank you for the opportunities you have created for me to grow not only as an educator but also as a researcher.

I would also like to recognize Dr. Patima Silsupadol and Dr. Kristen Mooney for their assistance in the analysis process of this project. Patima, thank you for stepping into the role as my expert validator and for providing the much-appreciated physical therapy perspective to my work. Kristen, thank you for serving as my co-coder throughout the analysis process. I am indebted to you for taking on this role given your own work and academic demands. I am honored to call you both colleagues and friends. Additionally, I would like to thank Dr. Myra Sabir for being the first person I approached regarding this work to share in my excitement about it. Myra, without you I am not sure that I would have pursued this line of research. Thank you for taking the first meeting with me and for connecting me with Sarah.

I would like to acknowledge my friends and colleagues in the CRA program, especially my Quant 2 lab group - Erin, Gauri, and Kelley. You three have lifted me up and helped push me through some of the most challenging times in this program. I am blessed to have had the opportunity to work with you all and thankful to call you friends. I have no doubt that you all will continue to achieve excellence on your journeys. I would also like to thank the Fyzigals for their constant support throughout my doctoral journey and for oftentimes putting me on an undeserving pedestal. You ladies have been my cheerleaders and told me to push through when I did not think I could anymore. Cara, thank you for your check-ins and willingness to help in whatever way you can. You have shown me when there's a will there's a way. You have inspired me to never give up, I am honored to call you a friend.

I want to thank my family and friends for their love and support throughout this process. To my parents and sisters, thank you for believing in me when I found it hard to do it for myself. Thank you for reminding me to be kind to myself and to trust the process. Mom and Dad, you have been my biggest supporters from day one and have instilled in me the values that guide my life's work. Thank you for taking every panicked phone call and listening to my highs and lows. I would also like to extend a special thanks to my Dad and Nana for inspiring this project. To my in-laws, thank you for your love and support throughout this journey, and for reminding me that no matter the outcome I will still be their favorite daughter-in-law.

Lastly, thank you to my loving husband, Chris. I truly would not have been able to complete this journey without your love and support. Thank you for understanding my extended work hours to finish this project and always making sure I had what I needed to be successful. Thank you for believing in me that I will accomplish my goals both professionally and academically. I love you and cannot thank you enough for the sacrifices you have made and the extra work and emotional load you have taken on to help me through this process.

I would also like to acknowledge the College of Community and Public Affairs at Binghamton University for granting me a CCPA Dissertation Research Award. This award provided the funds to carry out this research project.

Table of Contents

List of Tables xiii

List of Figures xiv

Chapter 1: Introduction 1

    Background 2

    Definition of Terms 7

    Purpose of the Study 9

    Importance of the Study 9

    Theoretical Frameworks 10

    Research Questions 12

    Overview of Research Design 13

Chapter 2: Literature Review 16

    Theoretical Considerations 17

        Biopsychosocial Model 17

        Relational Turbulence Theory 24

        Synthesis of Theoretical Frameworks 25

    Fall Trends Over the Last 10 Years 26

    Considerations for Fear of Falling 29

        Biological Factors 30

        Psychological Factors 32

        Social Factors 33

    Considerations for Caregiver Concern for Falls 34

    Caregiver-Care Recipient Dyad Considerations 36

    Gaps in Literature 40

Chapter 3: Methods 42

    Research Questions 42

    Research Design 45

    Sampling Procedures 47

    Data Collection 52

    Procedure 56

    Data Analysis Strategy 58

    Improving Rigor of the Study 61

    Researcher Role and Positionality 62

Chapter 4: Results 67

    Participant Profiles 67

    Major Findings 73

        Care Recipient Experiences 73

        Caregiver Experiences 84

        Dyad Experiences 93

    The Essence of Fear of Falling 101

Chapter 5: Discussion 102

    Understanding the Essence of Fear of Falling 104

        Essence of Care Recipient Experiences 105

        Essence of Caregiver Experiences 109

        Essence of Dyad Experiences 113

    Relational Considerations for Fear of Falling 115

    Implications 118

        Clinical Implications for Physical Therapists 119

        Implications for Interprofessional Collaboration 121

    Limitations 121

        Theoretical Limitations 122

        Methodological Limitations 122

        Bias 125

Suggestions for Future Work 126
Conclusions 127

List of Tables

Table 1 27

Table 2 72

Table 3 73

List of Figures

Figure 1 19

Figure 2 30

Figure 3 41

Figure 4 74

Figure 5 88

Figure 6 127

Chapter 1: Introduction

Fear of falling (FoF) has been a topic of interest in rehabilitation and nursing literature since the 1980s (MacKay et al., 2021; Murphy & Issacs, 1982; Tinetti et al., 1990; Tinetti & Powell, 1993; Vellas et al., 1997). Murphy and Issacs (1982) first identified the concept of FoF as "post-fall syndrome" (p. 265). Post-fall syndrome was described as the clinical presentation displayed by an individual following a fall which relates to gait abnormalities and fear of walking or standing unsupported (Murphy & Issacs, 1982). Post-fall syndrome symptoms can range from moderate to severe (Murphy & Issacs, 1982). Since that time, researchers have refined the definition of FoF to capture the fear and avoidance of activities that one remains capable of performing (MacKay et al., 2021; Tinetti & Powell, 1993). Existing literature has sought to focus on the definition and measurement of FoF (Bower et al., 2015; Delebaere et al., 2010a; Hauer et al., 2010; Helbostad et al., 2010; MacKay et al., 2021; Tinetti et al., 1990; Tinetti & Powell, 1993; Yardley et al., 2005), identification of risk factors for the development of FoF (de Souza et al., 2022; Lavedán et al., 2018; Lee et al., 2018; Liu, 2015; MacKay et al., 2021; Öztürk et al., 2020; Vellas et al., 1997), and interventions for the treatment of FoF (Whipple et al., 2018; Zijlstra et al., 2007).

This phenomenological dissertation study aimed to explore the essence of FoF within the context of the caregiver - care recipient dyad utilizing a biopsychosocial framework. By exploring "the essence" of this phenomenon, the principal investigator sought to understand the vital elements of how FoF is experienced within caregiving dyads. Existing literature examines fall risk and risk factors for developing FoF within biological, psychological, and/or social/environmental domains. A special consideration for social factors associated with FoF is whether or not the caregiver of an older adult has concern about the older adult falling (Ang et al., 2020b; Yang et al., 2019). Exploration of the essence of FoF, within the context of the caregiver - care recipient relationship, has not been explored with respect to the dyad as a whole. In particular, this inquiry sought to inform the evaluation process for physical therapists who must often navigate this relationship while delivering care to address FoF.

This introductory chapter presents background knowledge regarding the phenomenon of FoF, as well as the relevance of how it impacts older adults and their caregivers. Key terminology for the study of FoF is provided with definitions. The purpose and significance of this study, and the theoretical frameworks guiding the inquiry are also explored. The chapter concludes with a brief overview of the dissertation study.

Background

An estimated 37.3 million individuals fall severely enough to warrant medical attention every year (World Health Organization [WHO], 2021). The WHO (2021) defines a fall as "… an event which results in a person coming to rest inadvertently on the ground or floor or other lower level" (par. 1). Falls are named as the second leading cause of accidental death worldwide, and adults over the age of 60 have a higher incidence of falling than the general adult population (Centers for Disease Control and Prevention

[CDC], 2020; WHO, 2021). Sources vary in their definition of older adults as it relates to falls. The CDC (2022a) identifies those over the age of 65 as "older adults" when it pertains to fall statistics, whereas the WHO (2021) identifies individuals over the age of 60 as being more at risk for falls. For the purposes of this inquiry, older adults were identified as individuals aged 65 and older, which is consistent with the CDC definition of older adults in the United States where this study took place.

The CDC (2020) estimates that one in four older adults fall annually. Following a fall, physical injuries account for just one facet of recovery. When an older adult falls, they are also increasingly likely to become fearful of falling, which has significant implications for quality of life and risk for additional falls (CDC, 2020). Prevalence estimates suggest that 41.5%-96.7% of older adults develop FoF at some point in their lifespan (de Souza et al., 2022; Lavedán et al., 2018; Lee et al., 2018; Öztürk et al., 2020). This wide variation may be attributed to gaps within the existing literature to fully operationalize what is meant by FoF, as well as measure the phenomenon with a singular scale (Liu, 2015; MacKay et al., 2021; McKee, 2002).

Current literature aims to identify risk factors for developing FoF (de Souza et al., 2022; Lavedán et al., 2018; Lee et al., 2018; Liu, 2015; MacKay et al., 2021; Öztürk et al., 2020; Vellas et al., 1997). These risk factors can be categorized into biological, psychological, and/or social/environmental domains. Biological factors associated with FoF include female sex, increased chronological age, muscle weakness, poor physical performance, poor self-reported health, visual impairments, arthritis, and osteoporosis (Lavedán et al., 2018; Lee et al., 2018; Liu, 2015; MacKay et al., 2021; Öztürk et al., 2020; Vellas et al., 1997). Many of these biological factors can be addressed by physical therapy practice. Poor cognitive function, which is considered in the context of biological risk factors for the development of FoF for the purposes of this dissertation, is also associated with the development of FoF (MacKay et al., 2021, Vellas et al., 1997). Psychological risk factors attributed to developing FoF include higher general anxiety, depression, and reports of increased daily stress (Lavedán et al., 2018; Lee et al., 2018; Liu, 2015; MacKay et al., 2021). Social/environmental factors associated with FoF are categorized into risk and protective factors. Risk factors include lower socioeconomic status, less education, being unmarried, living with friends rather than family, unease with the neighborhood in regards to safety in navigation of the environment, lack of social support, and a smaller life space (Auais et al., 2017; Lavedán et al., 2018; Lee et al., 2018; Liu, 2015; MacKay et al., 2021; Vellas et al., 1997). Protective social/environmental factors were identified as increased interactions with friends and family, greater levels of social support, and high access to neighborhood facilities (Lee et al., 2018; MacKay et al., 2021).

Given the multifactorial nature of the risk factors associated with developing FoF (Lavedán et al., 2018; Lee et al., 2018; Liu, 2015; MacKay et al., 2021; Öztürk et al., 2020; Vellas et al., 1997), the biopsychosocial model (Engel, 1977; Mosey, 1974) is a seemingly ideal framework to guide this inquiry. The key principles of the model rest on the idea that biology alone cannot explain disease expression, but rather clinicians should be assessing for ways in which psychological and social factors may impact patient presentation in a holistic manner (Engel, 1977; Engel, 1980; Lugg, 2022; Mosey, 1974).

An additional social consideration for FoF is the presence of a caregiver. Increased social support was cited as a protective factor for not developing FoF (Lee et al., 2018). There is, however, a gap in the literature that identifies the point at which social support may become a risk factor for the development of FoF. When an older adult requires the assistance of a caregiver, that caregiver can develop fear of the older adult falling (Ang et al., 2019a; Yang, 2019). Caregiver fall concern prevalence estimates range from 58-91% across both disease specific populations regardless of age and the general older adult population, which is believed to have contributed to the wide range reported (Ang et al., 2020b).

Much of the literature on caregiver concern for falls neglects to account for the perspective of the care recipient. Yang (2019) conducted a content analysis of the language used by caregivers and care recipients to describe FoF during semi-structured interviews. Findings revealed that both the caregiver and care recipient used words like "worry" and "fear" as well as "caution" and "aware" to describe the fear. Caregivers were more concerned about the care recipient falling than the care recipient themselves were, and caregivers used "we" when discussing fear where the care recipient used "I". This was the first study to investigate the dyadic relationship of caregivers and care recipients regarding their respective FoF; however, it did not provide an explanation of the complex interaction of the dyad and how their fears may influence each other.

Studies regarding FoF neglect to take into account how that fear manifests in and impacts daily life. Existing studies have been successful in identifying risk factors for the development of FoF amongst older adults. Yet, identification of these risk factors does not provide clinicians with considerations for the clinical interviewing process and evaluation patients presenting with FoF. Newer investigations have aimed to explore caregiver fear of their care recipient falling; however, they do not account for the perspective of the care recipient in tandem with caregiver fear (Ang et al., 2018, 2019a, 2019b, 2020a, 2020b). The essence of FoF within the context of the caregiver - care recipient dyads has not been explored. This dissertation study aimed to fill this gap within the literature, as well as provide recommendations to physical therapy practice regarding the evaluation of patients with FoF.

Statement of the Problem

Following a fall, older adults are at an increased risk of developing FoF (CDC, 2020). An estimated three million people over the age of 65 are treated in emergency departments for falls annually (CDC, 2020). For older adults with a history of falls, prevalence estimates of FoF can be as high as 96.7% (Lavedán et al., 2018; Lee et al., 2018; Öztürk et al., 2020; Vellas et al., 1997). FoF has been associated with impaired cognitive function, more rapid cognitive decline, increased risk of future falls, and mortality (MacKay et al., 2021). Given the significant number of older adults treated for falls, there is a considerable risk for individuals over the age of 65 developing FoF.

Due to the multifaceted nature of FoF, the evaluation and treatment of individuals who seek care should be aimed at identifying and addressing the pertinent biological, psychological, and/or social/environment factors contributing to their clinical presentation. Physical therapists must also consider psychological and social risk factors at the initial clinical interview process that may be just as crucial to address as the physical impairments associated with FoF. Physical therapists are well-equipped to address the biological factors that contribute to FoF. They are often less equipped to address social and psychological issues due, at least in part, to a heavier focus on the treatment of physical impairments over psychological ones within their professional training (Daluiso-King & Hebron, 2022). While cognitive-behavioral interventions are well within the scope of physical therapy practice, many therapists admit they do not use these treatments due to concerns about lack of formal training for proper implementation (Daluiso-King & Hebron, 2022). The lack of training for physical therapists necessitates the opportunity for additional disciplines to treat older adults with FoF and opens the door for interdisciplinary practice.

Definition of Terms

For the purposes of this investigation, the CDC's (2022a) definition of *older adults* being individuals over the age of 65 was utilized. This age was chosen over the age of 60 as defined by the WHO (2021) because 65 is typically used as the cutoff for inclusion criteria amongst studies examining fall risk and FoF in the United States (Ambrose et al., 2013; de Souza et al., 2022; Lavedán et al., 2018; Lee et al., 2018; Liu, 2015; MacKay et al., 2021; Moreland et al., 2020; Öztürk et al., 2020; Pereira et al., 2021; Umegaki et al., 2020; Vellas et al., 1997). In addition, the CDC is a United States based organization and the WHO is world-wide. As this dissertation study is took place in the United States, the CDC definition was appropriate. The definition of a *fall* followed that of the WHO (2021) as "an event which results in a person coming to rest inadvertently on the ground or floor or other lower level" (par. 1).

FoF is defined as "lasting concern about falling that leads to an individual avoiding activities that he/she remains capable of doing" (Tinetti & Powell, 1993, p. 36). *Falls efficacy* is the perception of one's ability to avoid falls during traditionally non-dangerous activities of daily living (Tinetti et al., 1990). The question asked of the care recipients and caregivers during the initial screening process regarding FoF is based on the definition of FoF provided by Tinetti and Powell (1993) as this definition lent itself to a yes/no answer. For the purposes of the present examination, FoF was determined by a self-reported "yes" or "no" reported by study participants when asked "are you fearful of falling?"/ "are you fearful of [care recipient] falling?" However, the standardized measure used to assess for FoF that was issued to care recipients during the first interview process is based on Tinetti and colleagues (1990) definition of low falls efficacy. For the purposes of this investigation, *caregiver fall concern* was defined as a verbal response of "yes" when the caregiver was asked if they have concern about their care recipient falling.

Caregivers (or care providers, carer[s]) are individuals who provide regular assistance to another person along the domains of everyday tasks, and may include formal (paid) or informal (unpaid family members or friends) services (CDC, 2022b). For the purposes of this dissertation study, paid caregivers were excluded from study participation. Paid caregivers were excluded as the measure that assessed caregiver fall concern has not been validated outside of unpaid caregivers. A *care recipient* (or caree) included any individual who receives care on one or more activities of daily living or instrumental activities of daily living, who lives at home, and is aged 65 or older. This definition of care recipient is consistent with the inclusion criteria used by Yang (2019) during a content analysis of the linguistics used by both caregivers and care recipients regarding FoF.

The everyday tasks that caregivers provide assistance with are often categorized as either activities of daily living or instrumental activities of daily living. *Activities of daily living* (ADL) include six functions that have been determined to be essential to daily life: bathing, dressing, toileting, transferring, continence, and feeding (Katz, 1983). *Instrumental activities of daily living* (IADL) are more complex behaviors that involve an individual's ability to relate with their environment (Katz, 1983). Examples of instrumental activities of daily living include: communication, shopping, food preparation, housekeeping, laundry, transportation, medication management, and management of finances (Graf, 2007; Lawton & Brody, 1969).

Purpose of the Study

This phenomenological investigation utilized a biopsychosocial framework to examine the essence of FoF within the context of the caregiver - care recipient dyad. Utilizing semi-structured interviews guided by the biopsychosocial model (Engel, 1977; Mosey, 1974), the inquiry sought to understand how care recipients and caregivers navigate their daily lives in the presence of FoF, by identifying the "essence" of FoF. Findings from this study may help to inform the clinical interviewing and evaluation processes for physical therapists and multidisciplinary teams responsible for the care of older adults seeking treatment for FoF.

Importance of the Study

FoF is associated with cognitive deficits, higher risk for future falls and premature death (MacKay et al., 2021). Given the high propensity for older adults to develop FoF, gaining an understanding of how older adults, and in particular care recipients, navigate their daily lives in the presence of FoF is crucial. Literature regarding FoF is largely quantitative in nature and does not speak to how the combination of biological, psychological, and social/environmental factors manifest in the daily lives of older adults living with FoF. This study utilized phenomenological methods to explore how older adults' daily lives are impacted by the presence of FoF, be it their own fear or the fear that their caregivers have of them falling. Currently, increased social support is viewed as a protective factor against the development of fear of falling (Lee et al., 2018; MacKay et al., 2021). FoF literature, however, has yet to identify if there is a point at which the social support provided by a caregiver can negatively impact the care recipient.

Specifically, this study explored how caregiver and care recipient dyads navigate their respective fears around falling by accounting for biological, psychological and social/environmental considerations. Uncovering a greater understanding of how FoF presents itself within this relationship will inform clinical practice, and in particular the evaluation process for healthcare providers caring for older adults with FoF. The findings of this study have the potential to inform clinical practice and demonstrate the need for a multidisciplinary treatment approach for older adults who have FoF. Additionally, the treatment process may be informed in terms of patient and family education. Clinicians must be able to maintain a balance between the needs and desires of their own patients and what the caregivers of those patients want and need. In addition to gaining a better understanding of how older adults navigate their lives in the presence of FoF, this investigation aimed to identify how caregivers can impact the FoF that a care recipient experiences.

Theoretical Frameworks

The Biopsychosocial Model

The current body of literature aimed at identifying predictive factors for the development of fear of falling consistently supports a multifactorial etiology (Lavedán et al., 2018; Lee et al., 2018; Liu, 2015; MacKay et al., 2021; Öztürk et al., 2020; Vellas et al., 1997). These predictive factors fall into biological, psychological, and social/environmental domains. For these reasons, the guiding framework for this inquiry was the biopsychosocial model (Engel, 1977; Mosey, 1974). The biopsychosocial model has been applied in the fields of medicine (Engel, 1977; Engel, 1980), social work (Berzoff & Drisko, 2015), occupation therapy (Mosey, 1974), and physical therapy (Dalusio-King & Hebron, 2022). The use of the biopsychosocial model heavily relies on the re-integration of the mind and the body where biological, psychological and social factors interplay to influence disease expression (Lugg, 2022). Engel (1980) suggested that the model was not designed to increase the demands on a physician to make a diagnosis, but rather as a framework to guide care. Since its initial inception, the biopsychosocial model has been utilized in the field of physical therapy as a means to guide clinical interviewing as well as improve patient outcomes (Dalusio-King & Hebron, 2022).

The biopsychosocial model was utilized in this investigation as a means to guide semi-structured interviews, as well as provide a priori themes during the data analysis process. By using this framework to guide interviews, this study examined how both caregivers and care recipients describe the way FoF affects the navigation of daily life. During the data analysis process, interviews were considered in the context of biological, psychological, and social/environmental themes.

Relational Turbulence Theory

Solomon and Knobloch (2004) investigated the transition from casual dating to formal courtship as a source of transition within a romantic relationship. They identified that relational turbulence is "tumultuous experiences that occur within romantic relationships" (p. 796). This initial investigation resulted in the development of the relational turbulence model. Roughly 12 years later Solomon et al. (2016) turned that model into the relational turbulence theory. The key tenets of the theory include: transitions are key periods of time within a relationship; ambiguity around the roles of the relationship in response to the transition complicates the relationship; and the uncertainty and turbulence associated with that ambiguity has implications for perceptions of the relationship. Knobloch et al. (2020) explored the concepts of relational turbulence theory within the context of caregiver - care recipient dyads. Citing changes in autonomy as the source of transitions, the authors suggested that uncertainty in the new roles of the relationship can influence caregiver and care recipient perceptions of their relationships. For the purposes of this dissertation study, relational turbulence theory was applied to understand how the relationship between caregiver and care recipient has been impacted by FoF.

Research Questions

This study aimed to explore the essence of FoF as experienced among caregiving dyads considering a biopsychosocial lens. The principal investigator sought to identify not only a shared essence amongst participants but also shed light on how care recipients, caregivers, and the dyads uniquely experience FoF in their lives. This study explored three distinct research questions. The first pertained to the lived experiences of care recipients, in particular older adults, in the context of their FoF; the second explored FoF from the perspective of the caregiver; and, the third explored how the dyad experienced FoF as a unit. More specifically, this investigation sought to answer the following research questions: (1) How do older adults who receive care experience FoF in their daily lives considering biological, psychological, and social domains? (2) How do caregivers of older adults experience fear of their care recipient falling considering biological, psychological, and social domains? (3) How do caregiver - care recipient dyads uniquely experience FoF in daily life beyond individual experiences considering biological, psychological, and social domains?

Overview of Research Design

This investigation utilized the principles of descriptive and essential phenomenology to explore how FoF is experienced by caregivers and care recipients of the same dyad. As described by Hallett (1995), descriptive phenomenology seeks to provide a detailed description of the studied phenomenon, where essential phenomenology aims to understand the fundamentals. The goal of this dissertation study was to gain a deeper understanding of the essence of FoF from older adults and caregivers individually and as a relational unit. By identifying the unique experiences, healthcare providers can be provided with recommendations for the evaluation of older adults with FoF Semi-structured interviews were conducted with caregivers and care recipients to examine how both individuals experience FoF in their daily lives with consideration of biological, psychological, and social domains. Inclusion criteria of the dyads included: caregivers over the age of 18, care recipients over the age of 65; at least one member of the dyad must answer "yes" when asked if they are fearful of falling (care recipient) or if they are fearful of the care recipient falling (caregiver); both caregivers and care recipients must provide consent for audio recording; caregivers must be unpaid and have the ability to communicate in English; care recipients must verbally self-report receiving care for at least one activity of daily living or instrumental activity of daily living, have an absence of severe cognitive impairment, and the ability to communicate independently in English. As part of the initial screening process a list of activities of daily living and instrumental activities of daily living were read aloud to care recipients and caregivers, both individuals must answer "yes" that care is received or provided for at least one of those activities. The caregivers were unpaid in the sense that they are receiving no financial incentive for the care provided. This decision was consistent with the work of Ang and colleagues (2019a, 2019b), as the scale used to measure caregiver fall concern has not been validated in paid caregivers at this time (2020a). Additionally, both members of the dyad must provide consent to participate in the proposed study. Potential dyads were screened individually by phone (see script Appendix A). During the screening process both members of the dyad were asked about their FoF or fear of the care recipient falling.

This investigation sought to interview each member of the dyads a maximum of three times. The interviews were conducted at the convenience of the participant, either in person or via Zoom. The first interview included the informed consent process, in addition to the completion of survey questions and a measure of FoF (Falls Efficacy Scale International for care recipients) or a measure of caregiver concern for falls (Caregiver fall Concern Instrument for caregivers). Additional open-ended interview questions were guided by the biopsychosocial model. Successive interview questions were determined following the completion of the first interview with the goal of creating a deeper understanding of participant responses. Interviews with each member of the dyad did not exceed two hours. The recruitment goal for this study was three to five dyads, four dyads were included. All interviews were audio recorded with permission.

The audio recordings were transcribed and edited using Otter.ai transcription software. Using the a priori codes of biological, psychological, and social considerations for the lived experiences of the dyads related to FoF, the interviews were initially coded using NVivo. The initial coding took place upon completion of the first interviews for all dyads. Additionally, a co-coder was utilized to assist in the development of the initial codebook. The primary investigator and co-coder met to discuss emerging themes and to develop a consolidated consensus codebook. Following the development of a consensus codebook, the primary investigator coded additional interviews, noting emerging themes that arose in subsequent interviews in order to generate a master codebook.

Upon completion of the coding process, codes were grouped into major findings under the a priori themes, and any additional sub-themes. After codes and themes were determined, one care recipient, one caregiver, and one dyad were selected to engage in member checking of the codes and themes. This provided a check and balance system that the chosen codes and themes accurately depict the experiences of caregivers and care-recipients regarding FoF. In addition to member checking, to improve the rigor of this investigation, themes were also validated with expert opinion.

Chapter 2: Literature Review

Falls and FoF have been found to disproportionately affect individuals over the age of 65 (CDC, 2020; Lavedán et al., 2018; Lee et al., 2018; Öztürk et al., 2020; Vellas et al., 1997; WHO, 2021). Additionally, individuals providing care to older adults may develop fear of the older adult falling (Ang et al., 2020b; Yang, 2019). Existing literature identifies biological, psychological, and social/environmental risk factors for both falling and the development of FoF (Ambrose et al., 2013; de Souza et al., 2022; Lavedán et al., 2018; Lee et al., 2018; Liu, 2015; MacKay et al., 2021; Moreland et al., 2020; Öztürk et al., 2021; Pereira et al., 2021; Umegaki et al., 2020; Vellas et al., 1997). For these reasons, examining the essential elements, or essence, of FoF within the context of a biopsychosocial framework is appropriate to understand how caregiver - care recipient dyads navigate daily life in the presence of FoF. Additionally, these factors can identify nuances in the nature of the caregiving dyad that should be considered by healthcare professionals.

The following sections outline the theoretical frameworks that guided this dissertation study, with special consideration given to the biopsychosocial model and relational turbulence theory. Biological, psychological, and social/environmental considerations are given to existing literature regarding fall trends among older adults. Current research regarding FoF is highlighted through a biopsychosocial lens. Caregiver fall concern is explored as a special social consideration in the development of FoF.

Considerations for the caregiver - care recipient dyad are also explored. This section concludes with identification of gaps in the existing FoF literature that were explored in this inquiry.

Theoretical Considerations

Biopsychosocial Model

Engel (1977) proposed the biopsychosocial model, as it is known today, as a means to change the way physicians approach treatment of their patients. Engel (1977) stated that the biomedical model of the time neglected to account for the lived experiences of patients and the way that social and psychological factors can influence disease expression. The medical field adopted the idea that all disease was explained by the body's deviation from an established norm and that even behavioral ailments were rooted in altered "biochemical or neurophysiological processes" (Engel, 1977, p. 196). Engel (1977) argued that the biomedical model was reductionist in nature as it conformed to the idea that there is a separation between the mind and the body. With the viewpoint that the mind and body are two separate entities, there was a limit to which the biomedical model could be utilized in healthcare. Engel (1977) noted this and proposed the need for a new biomedical model. He referred to this new model as the biopsychosocial model, in which disease and disease expression were examined in the context of biological, psychological, and social factors (Engel 1977). Engel (1980) explored disease in the context of a two-person system, the patient and the provider; where the provider is expected to formulate hypotheses based on how and what the patient has been feeling, as well as probe the patient for more information to be able to test their hypotheses.

The biopsychosocial model has its roots in General Systems Theory. Engel (1980) cited the systems theories of Weiss and Bertalanffy to provide support for his biopsychosocial model. Paul Weiss and Ludwig von Bertalanffy were Austrian academics, Weiss a biologist and Bertalanffy a philosopher; the two worked closely on systems issues in biology complementing each other with their different academic backgrounds (Drack & Apfalter, 2007). Both authors have written extensively about systems theory in the context of biology, (Drack & Apfalter, 2007). Weiss identified that organisms are composed of systems that allow for locomotion, and Bertalanffy argued that organisms themselves are organized into systems and those organisms exist in their own environments (Drack & Apfalter, 2007).

Engel (1980) suggested that while a disease process is happening at a molecular, cellular, tissue, organ/organ system, or nervous system level; the way in which that pathology manifests depends on the individual person as well as how that person is situated in their relationships with other individuals, their family, and their community (Figure 1). In the example provided by Engel (1980), the ideas of Koestler (1969) are supported in that an individual exists as the highest level of the organism system, but the lowest level of the social system. This idea is also reflected in Bronfenbrenner's Ecological Systems Theory (1977) which explains that there are five systems that interact with and influence each other which shape development, particularly in children. Interestingly, Bronfenbrenner and Engel published their respective papers in the same year identifying similar ideas about how an individual interacts within society but in different fields. The ideas expressed by both have informed the fields of childhood development, education, medicine, psychology, psychiatry, social work, and rehabilitation (Berzoff & Drisko, 2015; Bronfenbrenner, 1977; Daluiso-King & Hebron, 2022; Engel 1977; Engel 1980; Mosey, 1974).

Despite the fact that George Engel is widely credited with coining the biopsychosocial model, he is merely one contributor to a body of research that was ongoing prior to his 1977 paper (Lugg, 2022). More than twenty-five years prior Kenneth Kendler and Roy Grinker described phenomena that questioned the traditional biomedical model (Lugg, 2022). In 1974, an occupational therapist, Ann Mosey, used the biopsychosocial model as a means to guide treatment (Lugg, 2022; Mosey, 1974). Mosey (1974) rejected the medical model based on the needs of individuals seeking care from occupational therapists.

Figure 1

Engel (1980, p. 537) Systems Hierarchy

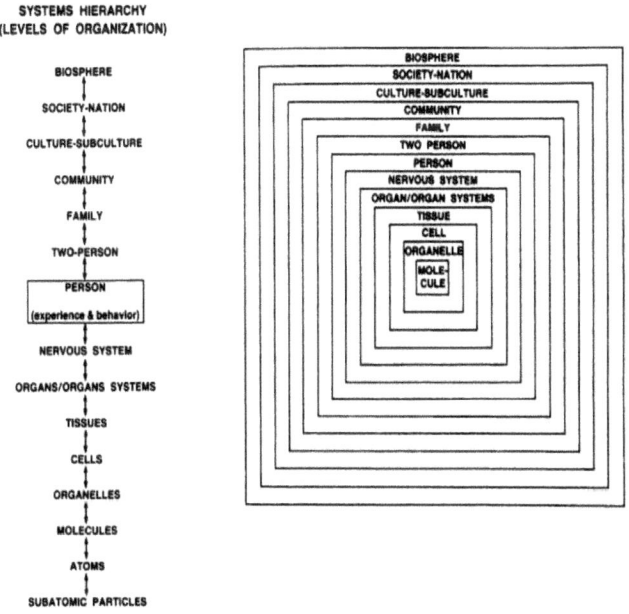

As a field, occupational therapists are interested in what happens following an acute condition, yet medical practice in 1974 did not allow for exploration of how a disease impacts function and disability long term (Mosey, 1974). The biopsychosocial model proposed by Mosey (1974) focused on body, mind, and environment without the assumption that the patient is ill or healthy. The biological aspect of disease is where occupational therapists focus intervention targeting strength, flexibility, and/or coordination; understanding "psychodynamics" addresses the psychological piece of the disease process; and the social consideration for the disease comes from the idea that patients exist within a larger society and, for that reason treatment should focus on living within that society with a chronic illness rather than curing the illness (Mosey, 1974, p. 139).

Key Tenets

The biggest differences between the biomedical model and the biopsychosocial model are that the latter is based on a systems approach, and it no longer subscribes to the separation of mind and body (Engel, 1980). The biopsychosocial model proposed by Engel (1977) posits that to deliver optimal patient care, providers must consider the integration of biological, psychological, and social factors in their diagnosis and treatment process. Drawing upon the principles of General Systems Theory, the biopsychosocial model suggests that while changes are happening within the organism levels, they do not become an outward problem until the individual becomes impacted (Engel, 1980). Once the individual is impacted their social system is affected as well (Engel, 1980). A failure of providers to assess their patients beyond the physical symptoms and impairments associated with a disease process can negatively impact treatment and patient outcomes. The biopsychosocial model allows patients to be seen as a complex puzzle in which any number of factors from age and biological sex to living arrangement and daily stress can influence how an individual experiences a disease.

Critiques

The biopsychosocial model has been met with criticism since its inception. The two most common are that (1) it lacks specificity and is too vague, and (2) scientific validity and philosophical content are lacking (Bolton & Gillett, 2019). Lugg (2022) utilized the work of Box (1986) to qualify the biopsychosocial model as a valid scientific model. He argued that to be valid, a model does not need to explain every aspect of a phenomenon, however it must provide some sort of utility in practice. Lugg (2022) utilized the example of mental disorders finding support for biological, psychological, and social etiologies. This investigation utilized this model because, FoF has been shown to be the result of the interaction of a number of biological, psychological and social risk factors. For this reason and the logic of Lugg (2022) suggests the biopsychosocial model as an appropriate means to guide the assessment of FoF.

To address the additional critique that the biopsychosocial model lacks testability, repeatability, and operationalization, Smith and colleagues (2013) devised a repeatable means for healthcare providers to gain access to appropriate biological, psychological, and social information at each visit. They highlighted a seven-step patient-centered interview: (1) setting the stage for the interview, (2) chief concern/agenda setting, (3) opening the history of present illness (HPI), (4) continuing patient centered HPI, (5) transitioning to doctor centered HPI, (6) overview and summary of HPI, and (7) completing the HPI with closed-ended questions (Smith et al., 2013). In addition to a seven-step interview, Smith et al. (2013) defined three habits that providers should utilize to make the biopsychosocial model repeatable. The habits included: (1) invest in the beginning of the interview, (2) elicit the patient's perspective, and (3) demonstrate empathy. The utility of the process outlined by Smith and colleagues (2013) has been investigated, revealing that there has been slow progress in the application of the biopsychosocial model in chronic illness (Kusnanto et al., 2018). The authors implied that the adoption of the biopsychosocial model in treating chronic illness has been slow due to impracticality of the model.

Utility in Physical Therapy

The biopsychosocial model can be utilized as a framework to explore many ailments that patients seek care for from physical therapists. The biopsychosocial model provides guidance for both patient evaluation and treatment. In a recent concept analysis Daluiso-King and Hebron (2022) worked to clarify the understanding of the biopsychosocial model in musculoskeletal physical therapy as well as explore its utility in clinical practice. They found that the biomedical model failed to capture the nature of pain and disability as the two often involve psychological and social components. When they applied the biopsychosocial model to diagnosis and treatment in musculoskeletal physical therapy, the characteristics of the model included: (1) a focus on diagnosis through clinical reasoning and physical assessment, (2) psychological factors included descriptions of feelings and emotions which impacted the patients experience with their pain and disability, (3) social factors related to job satisfaction, socioeconomic status, and unemployment as well as the psychological implications of those factors influenced how pain and disability were experienced, (4) communication allowed for more patient-centered care in which the provider could connect to the beliefs and fears of the patient, and (5) pain response was found to be affected by personal and social influences linked to a personalized plan of care. The authors also investigated how the implementation of the biopsychosocial model impacted therapy outcomes. Implementation of the biopsychosocial model led to improved patient outcomes and improved patient-centered care.

Despite these improvements, the authors found that there was failure of the application of the biopsychosocial model in clinical practice due to a lack of standardization, and provider discomfort with their training to address the psychological factors. The findings presented above indicate that there is clinical utility in using the biopsychosocial model in physical therapy, however there needs to be additional training of physical therapists in the screening and treatment of psychological impairments associated with musculoskeletal disorders. Given the potential for clinical applicability of the biopsychosocial model in physical therapy as a means to evaluate, diagnose, and treat individuals with pain and disability, special consideration should be given to the utility of the model when exploring the multifaceted nature of FoF. Noting the concerns of physical therapists for lack of training in dealing with the psychological concerns of their patients, the biopsychosocial model could be used to promote multidisciplinary action in the evaluation and treatment of older adults who have FoF.

Relational Turbulence Theory

Relational turbulence theory indicates that transitions are key periods of time within a relationship where turbulence can occur (Solomon et al., 2016). Ambiguity around the roles of the relationship in response to a transition complicates the relationship and the uncertainty and turbulence associated with that ambiguity has implications for perceptions of the relationship (Solomon et al., 2016). A relational transition is defined as a "period of discontinuity during which individuals adapt to changing roles, identities, and circumstances (Solomon et al., 2016, p. 510). While initially used to understand transitions within romantic relationships, relational turbulence has been explored in caregiving relationships as well (Cooper & Pitts, 2022; Knobloch et al., 2020).

Relational turbulence theory as explored in the context of caregiver - care recipient dyads implies that changes in the autonomy of the care recipient led to transitions within the relationship (Knobloch et al., 2020). For the purposes of this investigation, potential sources of transition in the dyads included a shift into the caregiving and care receiving roles. While not an inclusion criterion of this study, falling can also be a source of transition marking a period of increased caregiving need. Understanding the nature of the caregiving relationship holds special consideration for the application of this theory. Identifying what matters to members of the dyad is crucial. For example, spousal caregivers may be contending with transitions in their romantic life in addition to the level of independence of the caregiver. Cooper and Pitts (2022) explored relational turbulence in the presence of Alzheimer's disease and related dementias. The authors found that while most relationships will have a settling in period after transition, that was not the case with their chosen sample as the decline in cognitive status of one romantic partner kept the relationship in transition. This dissertation study explored caregivers and care recipients from the general community-dwelling population which indicates that there should be a time where the transition experienced by the dyad will eventually fall into a sense of normalcy.

Synthesis of Theoretical Frameworks

The biopsychosocial model was utilized in this dissertation study as a framework to guide data collection through semi-structured interviews. The a priori themes of biological, psychological, and social considerations of FoF were used to guide the data analysis process. In addition to serving as the overarching framework guiding this investigation, the biopsychosocial model also acted as a means to consider the theoretical frameworks, such as psychosocial theories of aging, that were utilized to understand the results. Understanding FoF in the context of biological risk factors has been well established. While the literature identifies social and psychological risk factors, existing examinations do not explicitly utilize theory to explain how those factors may influence older adults with FoF. Although relational turbulence theory has been explored within the caregiver-care recipient dyad, it has not been explored within the context of FoF.

Risk factors for falls and the development of FoF have been identified by the literature to fall under biological, psychological, and social/environmental domains. However, studies fail to report a guiding framework for inquiries regarding falling and FoF. Based on the presentation of study results, one can reasonably conclude that researchers are guided by some sort of biopsychosocial lens. Due to the lack of formally identified theoretical considerations combined with the lack of qualitative methods to examine falling and FoF, there is little guidance provided to healthcare professionals regarding how biological, psychological, and social/environmental factors influence the daily lives of the individuals they may be treating for FoF. For this reason, exploring FoF within a biopsychosocial framework with consideration of relational turbulence theory is crucial not only for participants to tell their stories but to also provide clinicians with valuable knowledge to give the highest level of care to these individuals. This dissertation study was unique in that participants were able to tell their stories of how they are impacted in their daily lives by FoF in the context of caregiver - care recipient relationship.

Fall Trends Over the Last 10 Years

As the world population continues to age, there is a need to identify who is at risk of falling among individuals over the age of 65 (CDC, 2020; WHO, 2021). There are a disproportionate number of older adults who seek care for fall-related impairments relative to the general adult population (CDC, 2021, WHO, 2021). For that reason, researchers have focused their attention on identifying trends and modifiable risk factors to prevent falls in older adults (Ambrose et al., 2013; Moreland et al., 2020; Pereira et al., 2021; Umegaki et al., 2020). Common limitations exist in the literature surrounding fall risk. The cross-sectional design of studies limits the ability for the authors to imply causation between risk factors and falling (Moreland et al., 2020; Pereia et al., 2021). Additionally, the use of retrospective design relies on the ability of the participant to recall certain things about their health which may not be reliable at times (Pereia et al., 2020; Umegaki et al., 2020).

The following trends were identified among adults 65 and older in the United states for the year 2018: adults older than 85 had higher reports of falls regardless of gender (33.8% reported falls); between the ages of 65-85 women were more likely to report a fall (29.1%, with 11.9% reporting injury from a fall); the ethnic groups with the highest reported falls were American Indian/Alaskan natives; reports of falling decreased as self-reported health increased; those living in rural areas reported more falls than those in urban areas; individuals who reported increased difficulty with functional tasks reported higher instances of falls and fall-related injuries; and adults who reported more physical activity also reported increased falls and fall-related injury versus individuals who did not report physical activity (Moreland et al., 2020). Ambrose and colleagues (2013) found a number of risk factors that can be addressed through intervention to decrease risk of falls, such as: strength and balance deficits, number of medications taken, and cognition. They stressed the importance of a multifaceted assessment to identify community-dwelling individuals who are at risk of falling to adequately assess all pertinent risk factors. Ambrose et al. (2013) noted that a screen could be as simple as asking the individual if they had fallen in the last year, then opting to conduct an in-depth screen if the answer is "yes". The previously mentioned risk factors for falls considered under biological and social domains, can be targeted by clinicians to change the underlying biological impairments and address social hazards that are increasing the risk of a person falling. An additional consideration for risk of falling is the psychological state of the older adult. Individuals who reported higher depression scores, were found to be at an increased risk for falling when age was controlled for (Umegaki et al., 2020).

While many factors are associated with fall risk, few studies provide recommended cutoff scores to determine when a factor becomes harmful. Pereia et al. (2021) provided cutoff scores to determine low, moderate, high, and very high risk for falls based on an individual's performance on a comprehensive fall risk assessment as well as other selected biological and sociodemographic measures. Scores on a multidimensional balance test (the Fullerton Advanced Balance scale) indicated that scores > 33 suggested *low fall risk,* 32-33 *a moderate risk*, 30-31 a *high risk*, and <30 a *very high risk* (Pereia et al., 2021). Lean body mass, fat body mass, and total physical activity levels per week were found to be indicative of low, moderate, high, and very high fall risk and do reflect factors that can be addressed by the appropriate providers to modify the risk of fall (Pereia et al., 2021). The authors also found that the number of health conditions reported by an individual in addition to the number of environmental hazards (both indoor and outdoor) reported by an individual were attributed to fall risk. Specific cutoff values can be found in Table 1.

With the exception of a few non-modifiable risk factors, many of the trends noted above can be addressed and modified with appropriate treatment. Physical therapists are well equipped to address the modifiable biological risk factors such as decreased strength and poor performance on balance assessments, additionally physical therapists can be useful in working with older adults to decrease their risk of hazards at home and out in the community. The presence of psychological risk factors may require treatment above and beyond what a physical therapist can provide. In these cases, referrals to trained gerontologists in the fields of social work or psychology would be appropriate. The trends and risk factors noted above fail to account for the presence of fear of falling.

Table 1

Selected Factors Indicating Fall Risk (Pereia et al., 2021).

Factor	Low Risk	Moderate Risk	High Risk	Very High Risk
Fullerton Advanced Balance Scale	>33	32-33	30-31	<30
Number of Health conditions	<3	3	4-5	>5
Number of Environmental Hazards	<5	5	6-8	>8

Considerations for Fear of Falling

After a fall, older adults can be left with physical impairments such as bone fractures, traumatic brain injuries/concussions, and decreased functional independence in addition to psychological impairments such as FoF (CDC, 2020). Among older adults who have fallen, prevalence rates of FoF vary significantly, with the highest prevalence estimates of fallers being >95%. Prevalence rates of fallers reporting FoF range from 25.1% to 96.7% (Lavedán et al., 2018; Lee et al., 2018; Vellas et al., 1997). These significant differences in the prevalence rates of FoF have to do with studies citing different measurement techniques (Mackay et al., 2021). More recent prevalence estimates for individuals who have fallen and report FoF are 50.1%, versus 27% for non-fallers who report FoF (Öztürk et al., 2020). The literature on FoF consistently reports multifactorial etiology encompassing biological, psychological, and social/environmental risk factors (Lavedán et al., 2018; Lee et al., 2018; Liu, 2015; MacKay et al., 2021; Öztürk et al., 2020; Vellas et al., 1997). In addition to identifying risk factors for developing FoF, researchers have also focused their efforts on treatments (Whipple et al., 2018; Zijlstra et al., 2007) as well as ways to measure FoF (Bower et al., 2015; Delbaere et al., 2010; Hauer et al., 2010; Helbostad et al., 2010; MacKay et al., 2021; Tinetti et al., 1990; Yardley et al., 2005). The focus of the following sections is on identification of the biological, psychological, and social/environmental factors that have been shown to contribute to FoF in individuals over age 65 (Figure 2).

Figure 2

Biological, Psychological, and Social Risk Factors for Fear of Falling

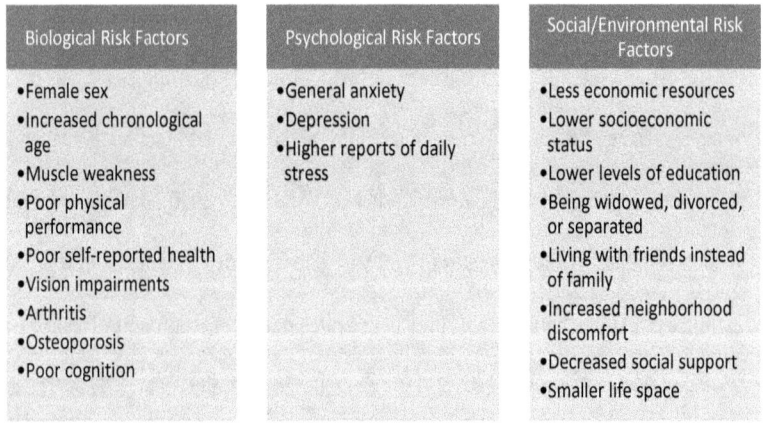

Biological Factors

Similar to falling, FoF is more likely to occur in women, individuals of advanced age, and those with increased muscle weakness/poorer physical performance (Lavedán et al., 2018; Liu, 2015; MacKay et al., 2021; Öztürk et al., 2020; Vellas et al., 1997). Additional biological factors include worse self-reported health, vision issues, arthritis, and osteoporosis (Lee et al., 2018; Liu, 2015). Cognitive status has also been considered a biological risk factor linked to developing fear of falling. Individuals who report fear of falling were found to have lower scores on cognitive assessments, such as the Mini Mental Status Exam (MMSE) and Montreal Cognitive Assessment (MoCA) (MacKay, 2021; Vellas et al., 1997).

Of the potential biological factors that are shown to influence the development of FoF, many are modifiable meaning they can be addressed with treatment. This is of particular importance as having a FoF significantly increases the risk of having a fall (Lavedán et al., 2018; MacKay et al., 2021; McKee, 2002; Vellas et al., 1997). Clinically, the modifiable risk factors mentioned above can be improved upon with the end goal of reducing FoF. At the present time, literature on FoF is largely cross-sectional in nature (Lee et al., 2018; Liu, 2015; McKee, 2002; Vellas et al., 1997). The results of these findings have very little applicability to assess change over time. Lavedán and colleagues (2018) used longitudinal data to assess if fear of falling was a cause or consequence of falls in community dwelling older adults. Findings suggested that older adults who were afraid of falling had double the risk of falling in a two-year period, and that women were four times more likely to fall than men in that same two-year period. Interestingly, Lavedán et al. (2018) found that once sociodemographic variables were controlled for, the association between fear of falling future falls disappeared. This last finding speaks to the complex nature of fear of falling as well as supporting the idea that social factors can impact physical impairments.

Biological sex and age are consistently found as factors that predict both falling and FoF (Ambrose et al., 2013; Lavedán et al., 2018; Liu, 2015; MacKay et al., 2021; Moreland et al., 2020; Öztürk et al., 2020; Vellas et al., 1997). These factors are non-modifiable indicating that older individuals and women will have higher rates of falling and FoF despite intervention. There is a dearth of literature to explain why women and older adults are more affected by FoF. One qualitative study by Mahler and Sarvimäki (2012) investigated five women over the age of 80 to determine their unique experiences around fear of falling. The themes that emerged around fear of falling, however, were largely in the psychological domain.

Psychological Factors

General anxiety, depression, and higher reports of daily stress have been shown to increase FoF (Lavedán et al., 2018; Lee et al., 2018; Liu, 2015; MacKay, 2021). One could also make a case that cognitive status could be identified as a psychological risk factor, however the literature examines it as a biological consideration (MacKay, 2021; Vellas et al., 1997). There is a dearth of literature giving individuals who have FoF and associated anxiety and depression the opportunity to express how that fear impacts their daily lives. Mahler and Sarvimäki (2012) interviewed five women over the age of 80 regarding their lived experiences with FoF. The women in this study became rigid in their daily routines to avoid putting themselves at risk of falling, often restricting their life space. Life space is identified as the mobility of an individual within their home and community (Auais et al., 2017). A second theme with ties to psychological processes that was noted was "living the vulnerable body" (Mahler & Sarvimäki, 2012, p. 41). These women were coping with the possibility that they could fall in a vulnerable or undignified way, particularly in the bathroom, where they often rushed due to issues with continence which increased their fear and stress with navigating their homes. The final theme from

Mahler and Sarvimäki (2012) with psychological underpinnings addressed the idea of overcoming or succumbing to their fear of falling.

The psychological risk factors of anxiety, depression, and increased daily stress suggest there is a critical need for a comprehensive assessment for FoF in which multiple disciplines are consulted. Physical therapists, who would address many of the modifiable risk factors are ill equipped to address the psychological aspects of the anxiety and depression that may accompany FoF due to shortcomings in their professional training (Daluiso-King & Hebron, 2022). For this reason, consultations with social work and/or trained gerontologists would be warranted to address the multifaceted nature of FoF.

Social Factors

The social/environmental factors that have been shown to increase risk of developing FoF include: fewer economic resources/lower socioeconomic status, having lower levels of education, being widowed/divorced/separated, living with friends instead of family, increased discomfort with the neighborhood, decreased social support, and smaller life space (Auais et al., 2017; Lavedán et al., 2018; Lee et al., 2018; Liu, 2015; MacKay et al., 2021; Vellas et al., 1997). Protective factors for not developing FoF include increased interaction with friends and family, high access to neighborhood facilities, and high social support (Lee et al., 2018; MacKay, 2021). Some of the social factors listed above can be modifiable with both individual and community-based efforts to allow for older adults to better interact with their environments. Lee and colleagues (2018) identified that strategies to reduce fear of falling should occur on an individual and community level. Implementing practices to enable more adults access to these protective factors is a continual problem faced by communities at a local and national level.

Increased interactions with friends and family, and higher levels of social support were indicated as protective factors against FoF (Lee et al., 2018; MacKay, 2021). Research has yet to answer if there is a point at which those social relationships and interactions become harmful regarding FoF. As individuals age, they may require care from family members or friends to complete certain activities of daily living and/or instrumental activities of daily living. These caregivers bring their own unique perspectives on FoF.

Considerations for Caregiver Concern for Falls

When an older adult receiving care at home falls, their caregivers will often worry about future falls (Ang et al., 2018). This concern can impact the relationship between the care recipient and the caregiver in a negative way (Ang et al., 2018). Prior to 2018, research focused on this phenomenon in the context of specific populations such as older individuals with stroke (Kelley et al., 2010), dementia (Faes et al., 2010), or Parkinson's Disease (Davey et al., 2004). Ang and colleagues (2018) began the process to validate a measure of carer fall concern for the general population. Their work consisted of four phases in which they ultimately developed and validated the Carer Fall Concern instrument (CFC-I) (Appendix B) (Ang et al., 2018, 2019a, 2019b, 2020a).

Phase one of the work conducted by Ang et al. (2019a) included a qualitative analysis in which semi-structured interviews were completed with caregivers only. The analysis revealed eight themes, four of which were tied to influences on the caregiver's fall concern, and four on the management of the care recipients fall risk. This investigation allowed researchers to understand the concerns that care providers have regarding their care recipient falling among a general population rather than a diagnosis specific one. The four themes regarding factors influencing caregiver's fall concern were: caregiver's perception of fall risk, care recipient behavior and attitudes towards their own fall risk, care recipient's health and function, and care recipient living environment (Ang et al., 2019a). The four themes related to management of the care recipient's fall risk were: fall prevention strategies used, risk of preventing falls, support from additional family and friends, and support from the care recipients' medical team (Ang et al., 2019a). Phases two through four involved the initial development of the CFC-I and subsequent drafts based on expert feedback and pilot testing (Ang et al., 2019b, Ang et al., 2020a; Ang et al., 2020b). Upon completion of phase four, Ang and colleagues (2019b; 2020a) developed a psychometrically sound instrument, the CFC-I, that is able to measure caregiver fall concern. Ang et al. (2020b) found prevalence estimates between 58-91% for caregiver concern for the care recipient falling. These estimates reflect carer fall concern for patient specific populations in addition to the general population. Carer's fall concern was found to stem from the outcome of the care recipient's first fall, the lack of care recipient awareness and concern for future fall risk, and increased distress when the care recipient did not adhere to fall risk prevention tips (Ang et al., 2020b). As the researchers focused solely on the carer, there continues to be a gap in the literature regarding the lived experiences of care recipients who have FoF.

Similarly, Yang et al. (2020) validated an instrument to assess fear of the older adult falling. While the terminology is different from Ang et al. (2019b; 2020a), the phenomenon of interest is the same: the idea that a caregiver has a concern for the care recipient falling, that is independent of that care recipient's fear of falling. The work by Yang and colleagues (2020) ended in the development of the Fear of Older Adult Falling Questionnaire for Caregivers (FOAFQ-CG). Prior to the development of the FOAFQ-CG, Yang (2019) carried out a qualitative study in which the caregiver and care recipient dyad were interviewed separately, the aim of which was to perform a content analysis investigating the language used by the carer and care recipient to describe fear of the older adult falling. Findings revealed that both the care provider and care recipient used words like "worry" and "fear" as well as "caution" and "aware" to describe the fear; carers were more concerned about the care recipient falling than the care recipients themselves; carers used "we" when discussing fear where the care recipient used "I". While Yang (2019) interviewed the dyad, the findings provided support for developing the FOAFQ-CG rather than understanding the nature of the dyadic relationship between carer and care recipient regarding fear of falling.

Caregiver-Care Recipient Dyad Considerations

Over the last 20 years, research focused on understanding informal caregiving has increased as a result of deinstitutionalization and decreased length of stays in rehabilitation facilities (Baronet, 2003; Jeyatheron et al., 2020; Lyons et al., 2002; Ris et al., 2019; Ward-Griffen & McKeever, 2000). There has been a call to understand the nature of the relationships between caregivers and care recipients within the community setting (Baronet, 2003; Jeyatheron et al., 2020; Lyons et al., 2002; Ris et al., 2019; Ward-Griffen & McKeever, 2000). Roughly 25% of adults aged 18 or older report providing care to another person with a long-term illness or disability in the United States (CDC,

2022b). Providing informal care has been linked to caregivers experiencing higher levels of depression and anxiety, worse self-reported health, impaired immune function, increased use of medication for mental health concerns, and increased risk of premature death (CDC, 2022b). Overwhelmingly, the literature has focused on the negative outcomes associated with caregiving. The focus of the following sections, instead, seeks to explore the complexity of this relationship by considering the caregiver-care recipient dyad in terms of the nature of the dyad, as well as to investigate current recommendations regarding how the caregiver-care recipient dyad should be acknowledged by healthcare providers.

Caregiving literature has failed to produce one single definition of caregiving because many researchers look at caregiving within a specific context (Schaffer & Nightingale, 2020). This lack of formal definition has implications for the support that informal caregivers receive from healthcare professionals. Researchers have aimed to identify ways in which to make the relationship between healthcare providers and informal caregivers more successful in the context of nursing. With increases in the amount of informal caregiving taking place at home, the efforts of those caregivers are often combined with home care nurses (Ris et al., 2019; Smith et al., 2021; Ward-Griffen & McKeever, 2000). Ward-Griffen and McKeever (2000) identified four potential relationships between home health nurses and caregivers, all of which led to caregivers feeling exploited by the home health nurses. They identified the most common relationship as the manager - worker relationship in which the nursing team dictated how the caregiver was to care for the care recipient oftentimes in the absence of formal training for skilled tasks. Two recent meta-analyses indicated that relationship building between the informal caregiver and home health nurse is imperative to deliver optimal care (Ris et al., 2019; Smith et al., 2020). The authors indicated that informal caregivers want to be recognized for their efforts by healthcare providers and be included in care decisions regarding the care recipient. The role of at-home nursing as a third member of the caregiver-care recipient relationship has changed for the better over the last two decades. Where informal caregivers were once exploited, they are now being considered as key partners in the delivery of care.

Literature regarding relational change and therefore increased relational turbulence has explored both romantic relationships as well as caregiving relationships (Knobloch et al., 2020; Solomon & Knobloch, 2004; Solomon et al., 2016). Therefore, understanding who the members of a dyad are is crucial to the research process. Linger and colleagues (2008) utilized three case examples as exemplars of different caregiver-care recipient models. The first was a reciprocal care model in which spouses take turns in the role of caregiver in the presence of acute illness, which is characterized by mutual respect and turn taking. The second model involved multiple familial caregivers where there was no appointed primary caregiver. The third model involved a multigenerational caregiving chain in which the child of an older adult was the primary caregiver for their ailing parent, however that ailing parent was a caregiver for the children of the adult child. These models of caregiving and care receiving held particular importance for this dissertation study because the relationship between the interviewed dyad members with respect to fear of falling would be influenced by the nature of the relationship. For example, with spousal caregivers, both members of the dyad experienced FoF for themselves given their age, with the caregiver having additional fear of the care recipient falling. In cases where there were multiple caregivers with no designated primary caregiver, there were additional social influences at play because each of the caregivers may have different levels of fear of the care recipient falling. Understanding the caregiving process unique to each dyad is crucial for healthcare professionals to determine because that will determine who gets the support and training (Lingler et al., 2008).

As informal caregivers often take on major roles in the delivery of care, they often lack formal training on how to specifically care for the needs of a care recipient (Benton & Meyer, 2019; Jeyatheron et al., 2020; Lingler et al., 2008). Depending on the type of care provided informal caregivers are at an increased risk of sustaining musculoskeletal injuries themselves from their caregiving duties (Benton & Meyer, 2019). In one study, researchers interviewed both caregivers and care recipients following discharge home after a rehabilitation stay for spinal cord injuries (Jeyatheron et al., 2020). Both caregivers and care recipients expressed that the caregivers were ill prepared to manage the needs of the care recipient upon discharge as they were instructed very few times on how to perform very complex tasks such as catheterization and transferring. Caregivers expressed that they experienced injuries themselves as a result of improper training and fragmented follow-up care after discharge. Both inpatient and outpatient providers should be adequately training caregivers who accompany care recipients on the safe management of the FoF.

Gaps in Literature

As the current literature regarding FoF stands, there is an absence of clear theoretical frameworks guiding inquiry, despite the fact that there has been overwhelming support for multifaceted risk factors for the development of FoF. In addition, qualitative methodology is largely missing from the FoF literature. While biological, psychological, and social risk factors for the development of FoF have been identified, the way in which these factors interact to manifest within the daily lives of older adults has not been explicitly investigated. This has led to a lack of guidance for healthcare professionals who treat individuals with FoF. Finally, FoF literature has yet to identify a point at which increased social interaction may change from a protective factor to a risk factor in the development of FoF. This dissertation study aimed to address these gaps utilizing descriptive and essential phenomenological principles through semi-structured interviews in which FoF is explored within the context of the caregiver - care recipient dyad. This research design allowed both caregivers and care recipients to share how their daily lives are shaped by the presence of fear of falling with consideration for biological, psychological, and social factors (Figure 3). Additionally, this dissertation study contributes to the growing body of literature regarding understanding the relationship between informal caregivers and care recipients and how that relationship needs to be addressed and nurtured within the context of physical therapy.

Figure 3

Conceptual Model for Proposed Dissertation Study

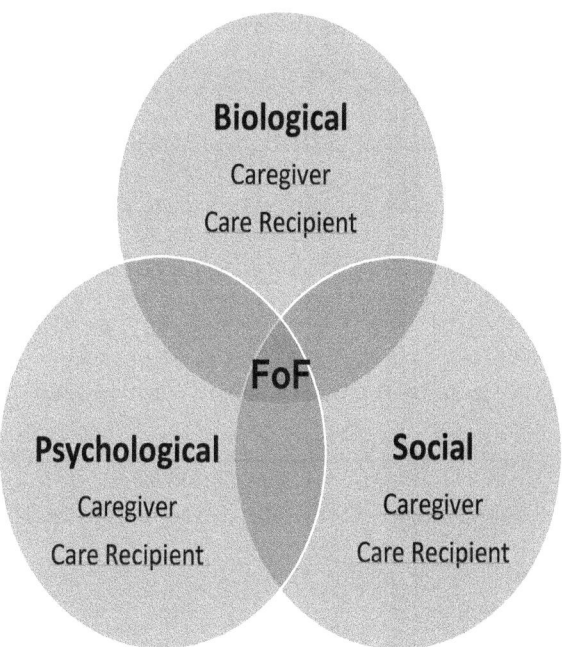

Chapter 3: Methods

Existing literature identifies biological, psychological, and social/environmental risk factors for the development of FoF (Lavedán et al., 2018; Lee et al., 2018; Liu, 2015; MacKay et al., 2021; Öztürk et al., 2020; Vellas et al., 1997). Additional inquiries have explored the concept of caregiver fear of their care recipient falling (Ang et al., 2020b; Yang 2019). FoF literature is largely quantitative in nature, and existing qualitative inquiries have only explored the experiences of caregivers or care recipients in isolation (Ang et al., 2019a; Mahler & Sarvimäki, 2012). Yang (2019) was the first to interview caregivers and care recipients of the same dyad to inform the development of a measure to assess caregiver fear of the older adult falling. To date, no studies have explored the essence of FoF within the context of the caregiver - care recipient dyad. Due to this lack of understanding of how FoF impacts caregivers and care recipients in their daily life experiences, there has been little guidance provided to health care professionals regarding the evaluation process of individuals with FoF beyond the physical impairments. This investigation utilized a qualitative phenomenological approach to explore how FoF is experienced by caregivers and care recipients respective to biological, psychological, and social factors.

Research Questions

To address the previously discussed gaps in this literature, this dissertation study utilized the phenomenological tradition to explore the lived experiences of caregivers and care recipients with FoF. The purpose of the investigation was to explore the essence of FoF within the context of the caregiver - care recipient dyad utilizing a biopsychosocial approach. A three-step semi-structured interview process was utilized to explore the following research questions:

Research Question 1: How do older adults who receive care experience FoF in their daily lives considering biological, psychological, and social domains?

The risk factors associated with older adults developing FoF have been studied at length, revealing that biological, psychological, and social/environmental factors all play a role (Lavedán et al., 2018; Lee et al., 2018; Liu, 2015; MacKay et al., 2021; Öztürk et al., 2020; Vellas et al., 1997). Where existing literature falls short is in understanding how those factors impact the daily lives of older adults living with FoF. This research question aims to identify the ways that care recipients are affected by FoF both in their homes and as they navigate the community. Gaining a deeper understanding of how daily life is shaped by FoF will provide clinicians with additional considerations for the clinical evaluation process and may indicate that FoF is best addressed with a multidisciplinary team of practitioners.

Research Question 2: How do caregivers of older adults experience fear of their care recipient falling considering biological, psychological, and social domains?

In the case of older adults who require the assistance of a caregiver, that caregiver can develop a fear of the older adult falling independent of older adult FoF (Ang et al., 2020b; Yang, 2019). Ang and colleagues (2020b) identified three sources of caregiver fall concern: the outcome of previous falls, lack of care recipient awareness of their fall risk, and frustration with the care recipient ignoring fall prevention advice. Increased social support and interactions with friends and family members are cited as protective factors against the development of FoF (Lee et al., 2018; MacKay, 2021). This poses a unique social consideration for FoF, because existing literature fails to identify a point at which the social interaction a caregiver provides may become harmful rather than protective. By interviewing the caregivers of older adults in addition to the older adults themselves, this investigation aimed to identify situations where caregiver support may impact older adult FoF. This research question implored caregivers to examine how fear of falling impacts their daily lives in terms of their caregiving duties.

Research Question 3: How do caregiver - care recipient dyads uniquely experience FoF in daily life beyond individual experiences considering biological, psychological, and social domains?

Changes in autonomy have been cited as sources of turbulence in caregiving relationships (Knobloch et al., 2020). As the level of care recipient independence changes, there is often uncertainty between both members of the caregiver dyad regarding each person's role (Knobloch et al., 2020). Attempting to understand how the dyad experiences FoF in daily life may help to smooth transitions and decrease turbulence within the caregiving relationship. This research question aimed to deepen the understanding of how caregiving relationships are impacted by the presence of FoF within the dyad. Understanding the nature and purpose of caregiving unique to each dyad is of the utmost importance, and has practical implications for physical therapists and other providers who are treating individuals who have FoF. By defining the role of the caregiver, providers will then be able to identify what supports need to be provided to best serve the care recipient (Lingler et al., 2008).

Research Design

This dissertation study employed phenomenological methodologies to the study design, data collection, and data analysis to examine how older adults and their caregivers experience FoF in their daily lives. Phenomenological inquiries rely on rich, detailed descriptions of the shared experiences of study participants (Creswell & Poth, 2018; Seidman, 2013; Smith & Osborn, 2003). Phenomenological inquiries are growing in popularity among nursing and health science researchers (Creswell & Poth, 2018, Renjith et al., 2021). The phenomenological tradition was appropriate to guide this investigation as the aim was to gain a deeper understanding of FoF through the lived experiences of caregivers and care recipients who must navigate it on a daily basis. Hallett (1995) identified various types of phenomenological inquiries. The two that apply to the proposed dissertation are descriptive and essential phenomenology. Descriptive phenomenology requires the researcher to ignore any preconceived ideas regarding the studied phenomenon while aiming to provide deep descriptions (Hallett, 1995). This study incorporated aspects of descriptive phenomenology to identify themes that illuminate the experiences of both caregivers and care recipients with regard to FoF. Essential phenomenology aims to understand the fundamental aspects of the phenomenon (Hallett, 1995). The components of essential phenomenology were utilized to explore the essence of FoF, aiming to identify what FoF means to older adults and their caregivers.

Central to phenomenology is the idea that researchers seek to study the subjective experiences of participants (Creswell & Poth, 2018; Hallett, 1995). Hallett (1995), identified two tenants of phenomenology: inductive processes to understand the phenomenon in a more general way, and positivism as a means to understand the nature of a phenomenon. As described by Guba and Lincoln (1994), positivism seeks to utilize research to determine the shared truth among individuals who have experienced the same phenomenon and typically utilizes more traditional experimental methodology. Park and colleagues (2020) further identified that researchers utilizing positivism as the interpretive framework use deductive processes to test a priori hypotheses. This investigation did not subscribe to traditional experimental processes to understand the essence of FoF. However, it aimed to utilize a priori themes guided by a biopsychosocial framework to explore the essence of FoF. Using a pragmatic lens to explore the essence of FoF was more appropriate for this inquiry. Pragmatism as an interpretive framework aims to "find solutions to real world problems" by understanding a reality through both "deductive" and "inductive" processes (Creswell & Poth, 2018, p. 35). The pragmatic researcher utilizes whichever methodology is appropriate to answer the research questions. Descriptive and essential phenomenology remain the appropriate method to explore the essence of FoF within caregiving dyads.

This dissertation study sought to utilize participant experiences as well as inductive processes to understand FoF from the perspective of older adults, their caregivers, and the dyad as a whole. Within the phenomenological tradition, a series of three semi-structured interviews were conducted with both care providers and care recipients (Seidman, 2013). Semi-structured interviews were chosen as they provide a framework to guide the participants while still allowing for rich descriptions of personal experiences (Britten, 1995; Smith & Osborn, 2003; Stuckey, 2013).

Sampling Procedures

Participants

Due to the rich nature of phenomenological inquiry, similar studies – in terms of either design and/or focus of inquiry – have had between one and 25 participants (Creswell & Poth, 2018; Denzin & Lincoln, 2005; Kuzel, 1999; Morse, 2000; Smith & Osborne, 2003; Starks & Brown-Trinidad, 2007). Sample size considerations in qualitative inquiry have also considered the number of interviews. Creswell and Poth (2018) and Seidman (2013) both advocated for a multiple interview process. For these reasons, eight individuals were recruited into this study for a total of four caregiver-care recipient dyads.

The inclusion and exclusion criteria for the caregivers were based on the same criteria used in the development of the CFC-I (Ang et al. 2019a), as the instrument has not yet been validated in any other caregiver populations. The inclusion criteria for care providers were as follows: (a)18 years or older, (b) a caregiver (self-selected by dyad) for family member or friend, (c) provide support for at least one activity of daily living (ADL) or instrumental activity of daily living (IADL) (Ang et al., 2018) and (d) self-reported having fear of their care recipient falling. Carers were excluded if they: (a) were paid caregivers or healthcare providers, (b) were unable to speak English, or (c) unable to provide verbal informed consent (per the approval of the institutional review board) (Ang et al., 2019a). In the event that the caregiving relationship involved multiple caregivers, the dyad self-selected someone to be the primary caregiver for the purposes of this study. The inclusion criteria of self-reporting fear of the care recipient falling was added because research question two aims to explore how caregivers experience that fear in their daily lives.

The inclusion criteria for care recipients were as follows: (a) living in the community and not residential care (community-dwelling), (b) 65 years of age or older, and (c) self-report of requiring assistance from a carer on one or more ADL/IADL (Yang, 2019). Care recipients were excluded if they: (a) were unable to communicate independently, (b) unable to walk independently (can be with or without a device) or, (c) had severe cognitive impairment (MoCA score <10/30) that could impact their ability to participate in the study (Yang, 2019). The inclusion and exclusion criteria for the care recipients of the proposed study were drawn from a number of sources. The scale utilized to assess care recipient fear of falling (Falls Efficacy Scale International) was validated amongst community dwelling individuals over the age of 60 (Yardley et al., 2005). The age of 65 was chosen at the cutoff as the literature supporting fall trends and fear of falling risk factors includes individuals aged 65 and older (Ambrose et al., 2013; de Souza et al., 2022; Lavedán et al., 2018; Lee et al., 2018; Liu, 2015; MacKay et al., 2021; Moreland et al., 2020; Öztürk et al., 2020; Pereira et al., 2021; Umegaki et al., 2020; Vellas et al., 1997). Yang (2019) was the first to interview both caregivers and care recipients regarding their respective fears of falling, and the remaining inclusion criteria in addition to including community older adults aged 65 and older is consistent with Yang's work. The exclusion criteria for the care recipients also echoes that of Yang (2019), with the exception of the verbal abilities of the care recipient. Yang (2019) excluded individuals who were non-verbal, which was seemingly appropriate given that the research goal of that study was to examine the linguistics of caregivers and care recipients regarding FoF.

For the purpose of this inquiry, both the caregiver and care recipient must have verbally consent to participation. Additionally, at least one member of the dyad must have verbally reported that they are fearful of falling (care recipient) or they are fearful of the care recipient falling (caregiver). Finally, both members of the dyad were required to consent to audio recording of the semi-structured interviews. Upon submission of the study protocol to the Universities Institutional Review Board (IRB), this study was deemed to be low risk to participants and written informed consent was not required for participation. In light of this, both members of the dyad were required to verbally assent to participation in this study to be eligible for participation. The study was approved by the IRB on October 26th, 2022 (STUDY00003799).

Recruitment Methods

This investigation required both caregivers and care recipients to be participants. Purposive sampling procedures were utilized until the desired sample size was reached. Purposive sampling was chosen because it emphasizes rich descriptions and focuses on data saturation by carefully selecting participants with a desired set of characteristics (Etikan et al., 2016). Given that the nature of a phenomenological inquiry is to understand a phenomenon through detailed interviews of individuals who have experienced the same phenomenon, purposive sampling has been found to be an appropriate approach (Creswell & Poth, 2018; Smith & Osborne, 2003). This dissertation study aimed to sample both caregivers and care recipients of the same dyad, where at least one member of that dyad reported fear related to falling. Shared characteristics of the sample included care recipients being at least 65 years of age and requiring care from a caregiver on at least one activity of daily living or instrumental activity of daily living. The caregivers recruited into the proposed study brought variability to the sample as some were spousal caregivers and others were children of the care recipient, or shared other relationships with the care recipient. All caregivers were over the age of 18 and provided support to the care recipient in the form of assistance on at least one activity of daily living or instrumental activity of daily living. This investigation sought to begin the recruitment process with one member of the dyad, and would then utilize snowball sampling to identify the other member of the relationship. Snowball sampling is a form of convenience sampling, where existing study participants identify other individuals within their own networks who fit the proposed inclusion criteria (Parker et al., 2019).

To gain access to potential care recipients and/or caregivers, the researcher received letters of support from two local physical therapy offices who agreed to allow recruitment flyers (Appendix D) to be placed in their reception areas. Two local community agencies for aging adults were contacted and the primary investigator obtained a letter of support to serve as additional recruitment sources. Upon approval from the University's IRB, staff members at one of the community organizations were provided with a description of the proposed study detailing inclusion and exclusion criteria in addition to copies of the recruitment flier to distribute. Due to the nature of their office, there was no formal area to hang recruitment flyers.

Caregivers could have included spouses, children, nieces/nephews, siblings, or friends and more. These varying demographics posed a challenge to the recruitment of care providers. For this reason, the principal investigator utilized an online support group for caregivers through Facebook, in addition to recruitment through the organizations listed above. The Facebook group's rules indicated that researchers were not to utilize members for research purposes. For that reason, the principal investigator was directed to an offshoot of the original group. The new group is another Facebook group where researchers are able to recruit participants following approval from group administrators. Recruitment through social media has been found to increase the likelihood that researchers target their desired population (Leighton et al., 2021; Topolovec-Vranic & Natarajan, 2016). This supports the purposive sampling methods detailed above. Recommendations for participant recruitment through social media include maintaining the privacy of the user and staying up to date on terms and conditions of the platform, (Arigo et al., 2018; Gelinas et al., 2017). Staying up to date on the requirements of the platform ensures that the researcher is not exploiting the users or violating policies.

After the initial recruitment efforts listed above failed to yield the desired sample size, the principal investigator widened the breadth of local community organizations to include a learning group for older adults as well as a local church parish. Email contact was initiated with the director of the learning groups well as the parish staff to obtain a letter of support to serve as additional recruitment sites for this investigation. In addition, recruitment allowed for the principal investigator to utilize their personal and professional networks to obtain the ideal sample size.

Participants recruited into this dissertation study were eligible for a 30-dollar Amazon gift card upon completion of the interview process. This was done as a means to thank participants for their time and the resources they expended as a part of the study.

Data Collection

While this dissertation study utilized phenomenological principles to guide qualitative methods, the measures detailed in the following sections do capture a great deal of quantitative data. The quantitative data was utilized to describe the sample of participants while maintaining confidentiality. This inquiry did not meet the ideals of mixed methods research (Onwuegbuzie, 2012), as there was no mixed analysis of the data.

Measures

Montreal Cognitive Assessment (MoCA)-Blind. The MoCA-Blind (Appendix E) was utilized as a screening tool to determine eligibility for study participation. A score of 18/22 on the MoCA-Blind indicates "normal" cognitive function (Nasreddine, 2010, p. 1). For the purposes of this study, older adults who score less than an 18/22 were able to participate in the absence of the previously mentioned exclusion criteria if they provided verbal assent to participate. The scores of the individuals who scored less than 18/22 on the MoCA-Blind were scaled based on the work of Melikyan et al. (2021), to determine the severity of the cognitive impairment. One participant had a hearing impairment, for that reason the MoCA-Blind was not performed, the principal investigator utilized the full MoCA (Appendix F) to determine cognitive capacity for inclusion into the study. The full MoCA has been approved for use with older adults and cutoff scores have been established to determine cognitive impairment. A score of 23/30 on the full MoCA was found to have a sensitivity of .83 and a specificity of .88 for identifying individuals with cognitive impairment (Carson et al., 2017). Severe cognitive impairment will be identified as a score of less than 10/30 (Montreal Cognitive Assessment Test, n.d.).

Demographics. Upon review of the informed consent document both caregivers and care recipients were issued an electronic survey and appropriate FoF measure. Electronic surveys were distributed through *Qualtrics,* the University approved platform. The surveys were different for both care providers (Appendix G) and care recipients (Appendix H). The survey distributed to the carers included socio-demographic information, in addition to the CFC-I (Appendix B). Additionally, carers were asked to utilize a Likert scale to rate how much they feel they help their care recipient with ADLs and IADLs. Items included on the ADL and IADL assessments include: eating, maintaining continence, transferring, toileting, dressing, bathing, communication, shopping, food preparation, housekeeping, laundry, transportation, medication management, and management of finances. The survey distributed to care recipients included socio-demographic information, the Falls Efficacy Scale - International (FES-I) (Appendix I), and a self-report of independence across activities of daily living and instrumental activities of daily living. The Katz Index of Independence in Activities of Daily Living (Shelkey & Wallace, 2012), and the Lawton Instrumental Activities of Daily Living Scale (Graf, 2007; Lawton & Brody, 1969) are two scales utilized by clinicians to rate patient performance on activities of daily living and instrumental activities of daily living respectively. As the scales are meant to be performed face to face, the items tested on each were included in the self-reported independence measures issued to both caregivers and care recipients.

Fear of Falling. Fear of falling was assessed amongst care recipients using the FES-I (Appendix I). The FES-I is a 16-item inventory where participants self-report their level of concern on a scale of 1 (*no concern*) to 4 (*very concerned*), higher scores indicate lower falls efficacy and thus higher fear of falling (Yardley et al., 2005). The FES-I has demonstrated excellent internal (Cronbach's alpha = .96) and test-retest reliability (Intraclass Correlation Coefficient = .96) (Yardley et al., 2005), and demonstrated better predictive power than the original FES (Tinetti et al., 1990). Since the initial validation of the FES-I, cutoff scores have been developed to identify those with *low concern* (16-22) and *high concern* (23-64), as well as *low* (16-19), *moderate* (20-27) and *high* concern (28-64) (Delbaere et al., 2010). Additionally, the FES-I has been validated in older adults with and without cognitive impairments (alpha = .92, Intraclass Correlation Coefficient = .58-.92), the FES-I was found to have good to excellent internal reliability (alpha = .89-.92) and good test-retest reliability (Intraclass Correlation Coefficient = .81-.89) (Hauer et al., 2010). Although the current investigation excluded individuals with severe cognitive impairment, the FES-I remains a valid instrument even in the presence of mild or moderate cognitive impairment. Scores from the FES-I were used to categorize participants in low or high fear of falling groups to deepen the analysis of study findings.

Carer Fear of Care Recipient Falling. To assess caregiver fall concern, the CFC-I was used (Appendix B). The CFC-I has excellent reliability (alpha = .93) and good construct validity evidenced by moderate to strong correlations (.51-.76) (Ang et al., 2020a). Additionally, the instrument was found to measure three different constructs under the umbrella of carer's fall concern (factor loadings .557-.809): concerns about care recipients health and function; concerns about care recipient's living environment; and carer's perception of falls and fall risk (Ang et al., 2020a). The CFC-I is scored on a 5-point Likert scale where higher scores indicate increased carer fall concern (Ang et al., 2020a). There are no known cut-off scores at this time.

Semi-structured interviews

Semi-structured interviews were conducted separately with caregivers and care recipients of the same dyad. This study utilized a three-interview model as outlined by Seidman (2013). The first interview explored the participants' experiences with FoF in their daily lives; the second called on the participants to describe their experiences in greater detail; the third interview involved participants reflecting on the experiences they detailed in interviews one and two (Seidman, 2013). Utilizing three interviews gives participants ample time to describe and understand how their experiences related to the studied phenomenon have impacted their daily lives (Seidman, 2013). In addition, it also provides the researchers with increased trustworthiness of the findings as the experiences of the participants should hold true across all three interviews (Seidman, 2013). For the purposes of the present inquiry, interview one provided time for the participants to get to know the researcher as well as understand the types of questions that will be asked. Questions during the first interview asked participants how they experience FoF within their daily lives. The second interview asked the participants to focus on particular experiences so that they can deeply describe how FoF impacted them. Finally, the third interview asked participants to reflect on how their experiences shape their daily lives. A detailed interview guide can be found in Appendix J.

The interviews were conducted separately to allow each member of the dyad to speak freely. Participants were able to select the mode of interview, either in person, via zoom, or over the phone. Interview two took place anywhere from three to seven days after the first interview. These were conducted in person, via phone, or via zoom, and caregivers and care recipients had the option to be scheduled separately to increase convenience. The third interview aimed to take place three to seven days following the second interview and was also scheduled at the convenience of the participant. Due to participant illness some interviews took place longer than seven days after the second interview. The timeline described is consistent with Seidman's (2013) three interview processes for phenomenological inquiry. The interviews did not exceed 90 minutes per person and were audio recorded (Seidman, 2013).

Procedure

Recruitment for this dissertation study began in November of 2022 and ran through February of 2023. Potential dyads were screened via a telephone call (see script Appendix A) during which one or both members of the dyad must have replied "yes" when asked if they (the care recipient) are fearful of falling or if they (the caregiver) are fearful of their care recipient falling. During the pre-screen call potential participants were questioned regarding inclusion and exclusion criteria. Finally, the care-recipient of each dyad was screened for cognitive impairment using the MoCA blind. One participant was hard of hearing, so the full MoCA was performed in person. Care recipients who scored below 18/22 were able to participate in the study if they were able to communicate independently in English and provided verbal assent to participate, and the score did not indicate severe cognitive impairment (Nasreddine, 2010). Both members of the dyad provided verbal assent to participate over the phone.

Upon completion of the pre-screen process, eligible dyads were asked to schedule their first semi-structured interview (Appendix K email reminder). At the time of the scheduled interview, the researcher reviewed the informed consent document with both members of the dyad (Appendix C). Dyads were required to assent to audio recordings of interviews. The interviews took place at the convenience of the dyad. The interviews began with a brief introduction of the study as well as inform both members of the dyad of the role of the researcher prior to obtaining informed consent. At that time, the principal investigator indicated her licensure as a physical therapist, however physical ailments and pain complaints were not to be the focus of the interview process. Upon completion of the informed consent process, both members of the dyad were issued an electronic survey depending on interview location (Appendix G; Appendix H), additionally the care recipients were issued an electronic version of the FES-I (Appendix I) and the caregiver was issued an electronic version of the CFC-I (Appendix B). Once all surveys and questionnaires were completed the interview process began with the care recipient utilizing the semi-structured interview guide (Appendix J). The caregiver was then interviewed with the interview guide (Appendix J). The order of interviewing was changed at the convenience of the dyad. Upon completion of the first interview a second follow up interview was scheduled with the dyad, prior to which the interview guide was updated to allow the researcher to ask clarifying questions and probe each member of the dyad for more descriptive responses based on the replies to the first interview questions. These second interviews were scheduled at the convenience of the participants. Dyads were asked to schedule a third and final interview, again to be completed at their convenience, either in person, via phone, or zoom. The interview guide was once again updated to allow the researcher to gain a deeper understanding of responses from interviews one and two. Each interview took no longer than one hour per person. Upon completion of the interview process, each participant was issued a 30-dollar amazon gift card.

Data Analysis Strategy

Upon completion of each interview, the recorded audio data was transcribed using Otter ai transcription software. The principal investigator then reviewed transcript files for accuracy, making corrections as needed. All participants were assigned a code to ensure confidentiality, and only the principal investigator knew which code pertains to which participant. Data was collected until thematic saturation was reached. As this study was a phenomenological qualitative inquiry, the analysis was an interpretive phenomenological analysis (IPA). An IPA differs from traditional thematic analysis in that some themes have been chosen a priori within the context of a biopsychosocial framework (Braun & Clarke, 2006). Additional themes were inductively determined from the data itself using the IPA framework (Braun & Clarke, 2006; Colaizzi, 1973; Smith & Osborne, 2003).

Interpretive Phenomenological Analysis

Colaizzi (1973) described a seven-step process for interpretive phenomenological analysis: (1) understanding the meaning of the data through listening to transcribed interviews, (2) extracting key statements, (3) generalizing those significant statements,

(4) formulating the meaning of the statements and validating them with expert opinion, (5) placing the meanings into themes, (6) integrating the themes to explain the phenomenon being studied, and (7) writing a formal statement. These steps have been echoed by additional phenomenologists in various ways, all of which begin with closely reading/listening to interviews, identifying specific statements, then grouping those statements into themes (Priest, 2002). Smith and Osborn (2003), identified four steps involved in IPA that take the researcher from identifying codes and themes to writing the formal report. This dissertation study utilized Colaizzi's (1973) seven step process.

Step one involved the principal investigator reading the transcribed interviews, both as a means to check for correctness as well as memoing the content to gain an understanding of the meaning of the data. The second step utilized a co-coder, who, along with the principal investigator, identified key statements that informed the initial codebook. The utilization of a co-coder can increase the trustworthiness of a qualitative inquiry (O'Connor & Joffe, 2020). Recommendations for the use of a co-coder indicate there should be a minimum of two individuals, 10-25% of the interviews should involve co-coders, and the process should occur early on in the analysis process to decrease the risk of faulty coding (O'Connor & Joffe, 2020). For the purposes of this inquiry the co-coder assisted in the coding of three interviews. Following a discussion regarding the initial codes, the principal investigator and the co-coder reached agreement on the initial codebook.

Following the development of the initial codebook, step three involved the principal investigator generalizing initial codes into more general secondary codes. In step four, the principal investigator generated meanings for the secondary codes identified in step three. Colaizzi (1973) identified that at stage four the generated code meanings should be validated with expert opinion. To validate the secondary codes, the principal investigator implored the assistance of a faculty member in the physical therapy department. This individual holds licensure as a physical therapist and has completed her PhD in Motor Control. She spent 13 years as a physical therapy faculty in Thailand where her research lies in studying falls in older adults. Agreement was reached regarding meaning of secondary codes. Following validation of meanings of secondary codes, inductive themes and subthemes were identified (step five). The inductive themes identified in the data analysis process were categorized under the a priori themes determined by the biopsychosocial model. These a priori themes include biological, psychological, and social considerations. Step six applied the inductively determined themes to existing knowledge regarding the phenomenon of FoF. The data analysis process concluded with the writing of the formal report.

Saturation

Qualitative studies often note that analysis and data collection cease once saturation is achieved. Very few actually describe how the authors determined that saturation was achieved (Marshall et al., 2013). Marshall and colleagues (2013) identified best practices for determining and justifying when saturation has occurred. The authors found that second-best practice was to cite other similar studies for their use of saturation. For the purposes of this study, saturation coincided with other phenomenological inquiries in healthcare. Saturation was achieved after all interviews of the eight participants were completed, which is consistent with Grant (2022) and Wells-Johnson (2022).

Improving Rigor of the Study

Lincoln and Guba (1985) determined four ways to assess rigor of qualitative studies including: credibility, transferability, dependability, and confirmability. Credibility involves processes related to establishing that the results of an inquiry are trustworthy, true, and believable from the point of view of the participants (Lincoln & Guba, 1985). To address the credibility of the dissertation study, member checking was utilized (Candala, 2019). Practices for member checking vary in the literature. Creswell (2005) recommended one or more participants be utilized for the process of member checking. Given the relatively small sample size of this inquiry one caregiver, one care recipient, and one dyad were selected for the member checking process. Following a verbal discussion with the selected participants agreement was reached with regard to the inductive themes and subthemes identified in the analytic process. Transferability addresses the ability of the research findings to be generalized to additional contexts (Lincoln & Guba, 1985). Transferability of the findings is a limitation of this study as the participants were carefully selected to provide rich and detailed insight into their experiences with fear of falling. The use of purposeful sampling decreases the ability of the anticipated findings to be applicable in a more general population (Taherdoost, 2016). However, utilizing purposive sampling procedures does allow the findings of this dissertation study to be generalized within the study of FoF. Dependability addresses the ability of the research to be repeatable under similar sampling and contextual conditions (Lincoln & Guba, 1985). To improve dependability of this investigation the detailed interview guide (Appendix J) will provide the basis for general questions to be asked in future research inquiries. Following Seidman's (2013) procedures for a three-step interview process allows for the data collection process to be repeated in the future, thus increasing dependability of this study. Confirmability is addressed by identifying if the results of a study can be confirmed by other researchers (Lincoln & Guba, 1985). To ensure confirmability of findings this inquiry utilized a co-coder in addition to validating themes in the analysis process with expert opinion. The credentials of the individual who will be utilized to provide expert opinion are detailed above. The co-coder who assisted with the initial coding process, strengthens confirmability as she too is a licensed physical therapist with extensive training working with individuals who have neurological deficits. Additionally, the co-coder is a fellow doctoral student pursuing a qualitative dissertation.

Researcher Role and Positionality

I have been a licensed physical therapist for the last seven years. I have also been a granddaughter for the last 31 years. The interaction of these two facets of my life have set the stage for my line of inquiry. I grew up an able bodied, middle-class, white woman with two college-educated working parents. At the age of three, my parents purchased my father's childhood home from my grandmother (Nana), and she, as I like to say, came with the house. Until I left for college at age 18, I lived in a multi-generational household. When I first began a PhD program, I had no idea how my formal training as a physical therapist and my upbringing in a multi-generational household would be the guiding forces throughout my program completion.

From a young age I wanted to become a physical therapist. This was not because I was ever injured and saw a physical therapist myself, but because I researched it for career day in middle school and it seemed like a fun job. The summer before my senior year of high school I remember a conversation I had with my mom that started with a simple question of "What do you think you want to study in college?" and ended with "You can't pick a career off of a research project you did five years ago!" My response was something along the lines of "watch me!" The next summer, I was off to a six-year Doctor of Physical Therapy (DPT) program. My first three undergraduate years were spent at a small private liberal arts college. The following three years were spent as a DPT student at the same college.

During my time in school, I participated in pro-bono clinics, where the physical therapy students would provide care to students, faculty, and community members who might not otherwise be able to receive care. Those experiences shaped me into the provider I am today. I learned compassion, altruism, and that I should always balance the needs, wants, and expectations of my clients with best practice. When I was ready to join the workforce, I felt I could do so with patient-centered care at the forefront of my practice.

I started my clinical practice at 23 years old. I distinctly remember greeting my first new patient that I would treat without any guidance from my co-workers. I walked out of my office with my shiny new name tag that said "Dr. Molly Higgins, DPT" and greeted the patient (a male in his mid-70's). The first thing he asked was if I was looking for my mom? To which he followed up, "I have socks older than you." I was shocked and deflated after that interaction and thought, what else can I do to prove myself.

This was the first, among many times that I would experience ageism in my professional practice. My own experiences of ageism made me more acutely aware of how it manifests in the profession of physical therapy. Throughout my years in clinical practice, the poor treatment of older adults in health care became abundantly clear to me. Over the last three years in particular, I have taken an interest in bettering my clinical practice to serve the needs of the aging population. I have found that when people are treated with respect and dignity, they become much more active participants in their own healthcare.

Three years ago, I was approached by a physician that I work closely with. He asked if I would be interested in going to medical school and then joining his practice. He noted how hard he sees me work and the relationships that I am able to build with my clients and that he thought I would be an asset to his practice. As flattered as I was, I said no, because I did not want to be a medical doctor. I knew deep down that if I did, I would not be able to spend one-on-one time with my clients in the same way that I do as a physical therapist. I told the doctor that my true passion would be to join a faculty for a physical therapy education program, so that I could teach students how to be a voice for their clients in healthcare. This led me to enroll in a PhD program so that I could teach in the future.

Being in the College of Community and Public Affairs, pursuing a degree in "Community Research and Action", my coursework has been heavy with learning about "-isms"- racism, classism, sexism, ableism, etc. What I have found is that ageism is often missing from the content, but that is where my passion lies. As I stated before, I grew up in a multi-generational household, I have seen Nana go from working full time to giving up driving. She is just shy of her 93rd birthday and the functional changes that I have seen over the last few years have been shocking.

When I visit my family, I have a hard time taking off my physical therapist hat. I am often asked to assess family members' limbs for pain. I have two distinct memories from the last three years that have shaped my focus for the present investigation. The first came in 2020 after the COVID-19 pandemic took hold. It brought my mom, dad, and youngest sister home full time. Prior to this time Nana drove herself to the store and to get her hair and nails done once a week; she carried her laundry up and down the basement stairs and came and went as she pleased. When everyone began working from home her independence was slowly taken, not out of malintent, but because my family members thought they were being helpful. I call my Nana once a week. On one particular call I asked her if she enjoyed having the house full again. She hesitated and said "oh yes it's really nice." I went into physical therapist mode and said "is everyone doing everything for you and they won't let you out of the house because they are afraid you will get sick?" She said yes. I called my parents and sister and said they should let Nana do as much as she can, or she is going to decline quickly. My Mom and sister agreed. My Dad is extremely protective of his mother and fearful that she will fall and injure herself, so he was a little weary of my suggestions. More recently I was home for a visit and offered to drive my grandmother to church. My dad told me to pull my car up the driveway so she did not have to walk as far, to which I replied "she has legs she can walk." My dad said "well it's scary," and I said "for her or for you?" This last interaction is what has brought me to the present investigation of older adult and caregiver dyads regarding perceptions of fear of falling.

In addition to inspiring my chosen dissertation study topic, the interaction of my upbringing, educational experiences, and clinical practice also has the potential to influence the analytic process for this study. My bias lies in the caregiver projecting their fears onto the care recipient and thus leading to decreased independence for the care recipient. I have made attempts to limit this bias by asking open ended interview questions to participants as well as utilizing a co-coder early in the analysis process. My analysis also included expert opinion and member checking of the inductive themes that emerge from the proposed investigation

Chapter 4: Results

This study sought to answer the following three research questions using a phenomenological design and a biopsychosocial lens: (1) How do older adults who receive care experience FoF in their daily lives considering biological, psychological, and social domains? (2) How do caregivers of older adults experience fear of their care recipient falling considering biological, psychological, and social domains? (3) How do caregiver - care recipient dyads uniquely experience FoF in daily life beyond individual experiences considering biological, psychological, and social domains? A series of three semi-structured interviews were conducted with participants, during which they were each able to speak to their own experiences with FoF. Simultaneously, the principal investigator was examining the experiences of each participant for commonalities across the experiences. After screening eight dyads, four were recruited to participate in the study. A total of eight individuals completed the interview process. The following sections explore the demographics of the participants included in this inquiry in addition to identifying the themes and subthemes that emerged inductively from the interviews. This chapters concludes with the identification of the essence of FoF as described by the dyads in this investigation.

Participant Profiles

The study sample consisted of eight individuals in four caregiving dyads. The characteristics of each dyad can be found in Table 2. Care recipients are named CR00X;

Caregivers are named CG00X; and Dyads are named Dyad00X. The participants were recruited from a number of sources across New York State. Per the inclusion criteria, all caregivers in this study verbally reported a concern for their care recipient falling. Three of the four care recipients verbally reported being fearful of falling. Note that throughout the interview process it became apparent that the "fear of falling" reported by the care recipients was more indicative of low falls efficacy as none reported the activity avoidance associated with a true fear of falling as defined by Tinetti and Powell (1993). All care recipients in this investigation had fallen at least one time in the last five years per self-report or per the caregiver's report. Three of the four care recipients had fallen at least one time in the last 12 months. CR003 fell one time in his home after inadvertently sitting on the arm of his chair which caused the chair to flip over. As a result, he sustained a head laceration and required treatment at the local emergency room. CR004 fell in her driveway, was unsure what caused the fall, but was able to get herself up and into her home independently. She sustained a broken nose and neck stiffness. CR002 did not recall that she had fallen; however, her caregiver (CG002) reported one major fall in the last year and several smaller falls in which CR002 fell getting out of bed. Per CG002, no injuries were sustained. CR001 has not fallen in the last three years.

The dyads in this investigation varied in their make-up regarding the relationship between caregiver and care recipient. Of particular interest was how the care recipients perceived the level and amount of care they were receiving versus how much care the caregiver felt they were providing. Dyads 003 and 004 had no mismatch in terms of the perceptions of care provided and care received. Dyads 001 and 002, however, had mismatches in the perceptions of care. The caregiver of Dyad001 indicated that transportation was managed entirely by himself, that a lot of help was provided to the care recipient for housekeeping, and that moderate amounts of help were provided for shopping, food preparation, management of finances, and management of medications. The care recipient of Dyad001, however, indicated that only a little bit of help was needed for food preparation, management of finances and management of medications, moderate help was needed for shopping, and a lot of help was needed for transportation, which was indicative of her belief that she was still able to drive if she needed to. The caregiver of Dyad002 indicated that there was total assistance provided for bathing, shopping, food preparation, housekeeping, laundry, transportation, management of medication, and management of finances. The care recipient of Dyad002 indicated that she was independent in bathing and laundry; needed only a little bit of assistance for shopping and food preparation; needed a lot of assistance for housekeeping, medication and financial management; and expressed only total dependence for transportation.

ant Profiles

			Care Recipient						Caregiver	
Age	Gender	Race	Living Arrangement	Marital Status	Education Level	FES-I	MoCA	Age	Gender	Race
85	Female	White	Single family home, with husband	Married	2 years of college	27/60*	20/30**	84	Male	White
91	Female	White	Alone, Single family home	Widowed	High school, 12 years	25/64	15/30	58	Female	White
84	Male	White	With wife, townhome	Married	Bachelors	33/64	22/22***	80	Female	White
87	Female	White	Alone; single family home	Widowed	Masters	20/64	20/22***	62	Female	White

typically out of 64, however one question was left blank. ** indicates a converted score from the MoCA-blind. ***Score ind. **FES-I = Falls Efficacy Scale International; MoCA = Montreal Cognitive Assessment; CFC-I = Caregiver Fa** nt.

Major Findings

The following subsections indicate the major findings of the investigation for the experiences of caregivers, care recipients, and dyads as a whole as they pertain to FoF. A full list of themes and subthemes can be found in Table 3. The themes that are highlighted below refer to the essence of the fear of falling for the care recipients, caregivers, and dyads interviewed for this study. The major "essence" regarding the experiences of the participants were identified as the themes that sit at the intersection of biological, psychological, and social factors influencing their fall concerns.

Table 3

Inductively Determined Themes and Subthemes of the Essence of Fear of Falling

	Reasearch Question	Inductive Themes
Care Recipient Experience	1	Threats to Autonomy Acceptance Maintenance of Independence Influence of Caregiver
Caregiver Experience	2	Burden of Caregiving with Respect to Caregiver Fall Concern Reasons for Caregiver Fall Concern Compartmentalization During Fall Emergency
Dyad Experience	3	Planning for the Future Limiting Burden

Care Recipient Experiences

Upon completion of the three-step interview process, the principal investigator understood the essence of FoF from the perspective of the care recipients to be highlighted by the theme: Threats to Autonomy. This theme encompassed the intersection of the biological, psychological, and social processes responsible for the care recipient's FoF (Figure 4), meaning that the FoF was a result of how the care recipients perceived that a fall would threaten their autonomy more so than being fearful of the fall itself. Three other major themes, which emerged inductively from the interviews help to further describe the essence of care recipient FoF included: acceptance of fall risk, maintenance of independence, and influence of the caregiver (Table 3).

Figure 4

Essence of Care Recipient Fear of Falling

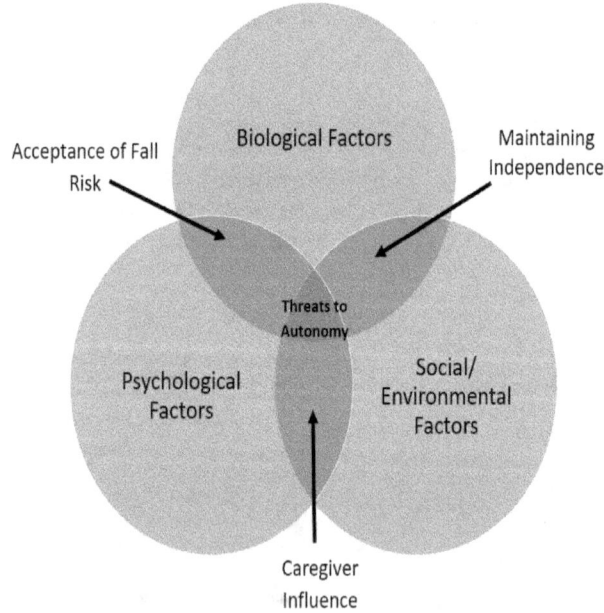

Threats to Autonomy

During interview three, the care recipients were each asked, "What does falling mean to you?" The goal of this question was to see how participants described the biological, psychological, and social processes that would be experienced as the result of a fall. While some participants noted the physical ramifications of a fall, others expressed what a fall could mean in terms of challenges to their autonomy and way of living. CR001 stated:

> I don't know whether I would break anything. You know, I don't know if I would break an ankle or arm or I think about what's going to happen to me ... And it could be anything ... it's rare if I fall and I don't get really badly hurt because I'm kind of heavy for my size ... I think you know if I fall, I will hurt myself somehow and will need help.

CR001 noted the physical injuries that would likely accompany a fall and could result in a need for increased assistance, not only to get up from the fall but also more care. CR004 stated, "Well it might mean I'd better get out of the house. I'm not really alone that much. Except for when I'm at home." CR004 expressed that if she were to fall again, she would likely need to move out of her home and into a place that is more accessible given her age and mobility deficits at the urging of her family. CR003 described the realization that he may need more advanced mobility assistance in the form of a wheelchair or scooter, and that this self-acknowledgement is cause for concern. CR003 stated:

> I convinced myself sometimes that I'm just facing the inevitability of it all. That eventually, yes, I'm going to probably have to transition into some other mode of operation other than just the walker, either a scooter motorized wheelchair or something like that. I don't know. And I don't know. I don't think it's going to be tomorrow, but it's out there somewhere. And at least, I think I'm thinking about it, and kind of vaguely making plans for that transition. That's the emotional...yes,

it's it would be an emotional not trauma, but you it's it the recognition that you're declining is a little scary.

CR003 reported that if he were to fall again, he would likely need more dependent forms of mobility which would be associated with a loss of autonomy as he would not be able to get up and go like he does with his walker. CR002 stated "Well, I have to try to call somebody right away to help me up…I don't even know my neighbors that well that I would call on them. I don't keep any numbers of them. I probably should though." From the perspective of CR002, a fall would leave her incapacitated on the floor unable to get up herself. She reported recognizing the importance of having social support that she can depend on to assist her in the event of a fall.

All four care recipients in this investigation identified that a fall would have some sort of significant impact on their day-to-day activity. CR001 and CR002 focused more on the biological or physical results of a fall such as not being able to get up independently or sustaining and injury. For CR001 and CR002, a fall was perceived to limit their autonomy because they would require assistance from others to get up. CR003 and CR004 indicated that a fall would threaten their autonomy in terms of mobility and living arrangement. CR003 noted having to rely on some other form of mobility would render him more dependent, because with a walker he is still able to ambulate has he pleases, with a motorized chair it would greatly impact his navigation of his home and community, he would require increased assistance from his caregiver to either manage a manual wheelchair or help load a motorized chair into their car or golf cart.

An example of a social consideration of FoF threatening the autonomy of the care recipients was found to be environmental concerns. Of the participants who verbally reported fear of falling, there were reports of environmental impact on fear of falling in both familiar and novel environments. Participants expressed that concerns about the environment can limit their willingness to navigate certain situations independently. Using self-management techniques, these participants were able to acknowledge the environmental sources of their concerns and adapt their mobility to prevent activity avoidance.

CR001 reported, "We don't go to any places that I can't hold his [CG001] arm, or have my cane, or both have a little cane and I hold his arm.". CR003 specifically noted the increased concern he has when navigating a newer environment:

> And anytime you get into a what I call a novel situation like let's say I'm going down to [physician's office], and I pull into the handicapped spot I've still got to walk 20 feet to get to the door, you know, I'm walking on the roadway. And so, you, you're looking, where are you going, make sure there's no hazard there that you're going to trip over or whatever. So, I try to stay in tune, probably at a somewhat heightened level, if I'm in an environment that is new, or novel or just unusual.

CR003 reported there is even more heighted environmental concerns in a new environment because is unable to draw on past experiences with the terrain to maintain his balance like he does at home.

Acceptance

As described by Kubler-Ross & Kessler (2009), acceptance is about learning to live with a loss. In the case of the care recipients for this investigation, the loss in question is a loss of independence associated with physical impairments and increased fall risk. This idea of acceptance intersects with biological and psychological processes being experienced by the participants (Figure 4). CR001 stated:

> I think I knew myself, what I was capable of anymore, and what I wasn't capable of. I think it was, you know, they didn't tell me you can do this, you can do that.
>
> But I just realized that I couldn't do a lot of things. It was self, self-knowledge.

CR001 reported being able to identify and accept that there were certain tasks she was no longer able to perform herself, without her caregiver imposing limitations on her activity. Similarly, CR003 stated:

> It's become part of me now, this, this caution, this thinking ahead. By necessity, you know, I don't want to fall again. So therefore, I tried to keep my mind focused on what I'm doing, and not just casually say, "Oh, I'm gonna just do this", and go off and try to do it. So, I do try to be a little bit more cautious.

Because CR003 is fearful of another fall, he reported accepting his limitations and is addressing them with increased caution to manage his fear. CR003 lives in a continuing care community where he would have access to higher levels of skilled care if he were to need them. CR003 expressed some uncertainty with making that decision and ultimately the acceptance of his physical limitations:

> How do I know when the time has come so to speak? You know what I mean? ...We've heard stories of people who say, "Oh, no, no, I don't, I don't, I don't need that. What do you, what are you talking about?" And I may fall into that category someday. You know of resisting it. Because of the, how do I say it? The reason we're here is because of that, because that the assisted living, or the skilled

nursing is here. And it would be will be, quote 'an easy transition'. It may be an easy transition physically, but maybe not mentally.

This care recipient and his wife (CG003), moved to their current residence for the purpose that it was a facility in which they had access to various levels of care to meet their needs as they age. In spite of the realization that a move out of independent living may be on the horizon he is not ready to accept it yet.

. The physical limitations described by the care recipients in this study varied from the result of an injury to general feelings of weakness and dizziness. CR004 had a fall last summer that resulted in severely limited cervical mobility which has impacted her ability to drive. She stated, "I can't move my head (since a fall last July). I have no movement." Despite significant effort in seeking treatment for her decreased cervical mobility, she still must rely on the assistance of others to drive her and carry out the tasks that require safe movement of the head and neck. CR001 indicated a general decline over the last five years or so which she attributed to advancing age. She stated:

Well, I'm a little woozier now than I was five years ago, actually. So, if I'm to fall, I'm going to fall now. Because I am not as steady on my feet anymore. I'm really dizzy, woozy. And that's old age, I'm afraid. I don't think it's gonna get any better.

CR001 perceives that she is more fearful of falling now because she is more unstable than she was several years ago, she notes age related changes that likely will not improve. CR003 cited an extensive history of lower extremity surgeries that contribute to his FoF in addition to age related changes. He said:

It's a result really of the diminishing of mobility in my lower left mainly lower extremities…When I'm trying to stand independently, it gives me great concern...But again, it's just the heightened awareness. I mean, it's also obviously age related. You know, I am 84 years old and having been a fairly active person All my life, the fact that I'm not no longer able to have the activity that I once had, causes me to have a heightened alarm or a heightened fear that I may fall again, I'm going to try real hard not to.

CR003 reported that he is unable to walk without his walker due to weakness in his legs that once they start to feel weak his fear of falling increases. Also notes age related decline. He is aware that his limitations are increasing his fall risk so he is trying to manage that by using devices to help him walk and be more aware of his surroundings.

Maintenance of Independence

The care recipients in this investigation expressed that falling would limit their autonomy and thus their independence. For that reason, they expressed the need to maintain their independence. In doing so, they utilized strategies to manage their fall risk to ultimately avoid a fall. Examples of strategies to maintain independence included the use of an assistive device and making modifications to keep their homes safer. These self-management strategies fall at the intersection of the bio-social factors influencing fear of falling (Figure 4). All four participants reported some level of increased caution when carrying out their daily activities. CR001 said, "I keep telling myself, be careful, be careful, don't. Don't trip on your own feet. And be careful that you don't trip on our kitty. And you know, things like that." CR002 similarly responded by saying, "I'm more careful going down stairs, and walking. And I think I am careful all the time when I'm out walking or anything because I don't want to fall." CR003 said that he has to plan his motor activities to maintain his balance:

> I try to do, just to think ahead of, just don't step but think, where are you gonna step? How are you going to step? So, I'm trying to pre plan every move that I make with the end, maybe not in the front of my mind, but at least in the back of my mind, this fear of falling and trying to avoid falling

CR001 and CR003 described how they combat their low falls efficacy when navigating their environments. CR004 described how she changes the way she navigates her stairs to maintain safety and prevent a fall, "I wear one of those alarm things. And, well, when, if I have a basket of laundry, I go down one step at a time backwards. I'll take a step and then I'll move the basket a step and another step." CR004 did not report that she herself was fearful of falling (her caregiver was the member of the dyad who expressed concern for her falling). By wearing a fall alert button and consciously performing activities on the stairs, CR004 reported believing she was able to alleviate the concerns of her family members to some extent, and keep herself safe at home doing the things she wants to do independently.

While CR001, CR002, and CR003 noted the use of an assistive device when walking both in the home and in the community CR004 stated she tried to avoid using one:

> My kitchen is sort of like a long aisle so there's something on either side. When I walk into the bathroom downstairs, I pass a long couch that I probably could touch if I needed to. I think I've been trying to improve my balance. By not, by not using a cane.

By not using an assistive device, CR004 reported that that she is maintaining her strength and thus improving her balance by not becoming reliant on outside sources of support.

She also noted a great desired to remain in her home and has made modifications to keep the home safe for her to continue to live in:

> Before I had a knee replacement, one of the first things I asked him [handyman] to do was to tighten the banister. And then after my husband fell, he [handyman] found a piece of wood or banister, whatever that he put on the other side. So that I have a banister to grip in both hands. And he's put grab bars up at the top. I think those are about the only things he's done to help make the place safer.

In addition to using an assistive device to manage his fall risk and increase his independence, CR003 expressed that he utilizes his walker as an extension of his sense of touch to navigate his environment. He stated, "And I use the wheels of the walker as a feel, you know you're hitting the rug. So, you just kind of just slightly (lift) up to make sure that you're not going to curl the rug back by pushing it."

Influence of Caregiver

To be included in this investigation, older adults had to be receiving care on at least one ADL or one IADL from an unpaid caregiver. The presence of a caregiver was found to impact the experiences these care recipients had regarding FoF along the psychosocial domain (Figure 4). The care recipients in this investigation were asked to reflect on what they felt the role of their caregiver was, why they think their caregiver is concerned about them falling, and how a fall would impact their caregivers.

The care recipients in this investigation identified that the reason their caregiver is likely concerned about their fall risk is because they have fallen or because the caregiver has observed some sort of movement impairment that would put the care recipient at risk for falling. CR001 and CR003 both fell where their caregivers witnessed the fall which they indicated as a major reason for why their respective caregivers were fearful of them falling again. CR001 stated, "Because I've fallen in the past. And because he knows I'm not sure footed anymore, you know, so I could see why he's worried he has every reason to be concerned." Similarly, CR003 expressed a similar reason for his caregiver's concern of him falling. He stated, "…Just observing the way I walk. The caution and the relative instability. That's why I think she's concerned and obviously she was right here when and when the other fall happened." Likewise, CR004 expressed that her caregiver has increased fall concern because she had fallen. When asked why she herself does not share the same concern she replied, "well they just see the outside results." She cited that her family dwells on the fact that she did fall and they see the end result of her being wobbly or at risk of another fall despite the work she is doing to keep herself strong and mobile with exercises.

Regarding the role of his caregiver CR003 stated:

It's just, it's an overall looking over my shoulder, so to speak. Reminding me of that, I haven't done something like, make an appointment with a doctor, you know. And so sometimes I have to be needled two or three times to follow through and do it. So she has a good tendency to stay on top of me, on top of my responsibilities to take care of myself by kind of watching what I'm doing and making sure that I follow through with what I should be following through with in terms of taking medications. No, I mean, I do all that myself … But it's just that she's kind of mother henning me if you know what I mean.

CR003 expressed that particularly in regards to his health concerns, his caregiver has to regularly remind him to stay on top of things. His fall and recent hospitalization were the direct result of a medical complication that he had not addressed despite his caregiver's warnings. As a result of the shared concern for CR003 falling, his caregiver's role has changed to make sure that he does not fall as the result of a medical issue that could be rectified. CR001 noted general family support for her increased care needs:

> I knew that they would help me. But they had no reservations about helping me at all. So I didn't find it a big challenge. Luckily…My husband is a good man. My daughter is a good daughter. I love them dearly. Because I know they, they care about me. And they don't want to put me in trouble. For any reason.

She stated that she believed her caregiver has no reservations about increasing his caregiving load as neither he nor other family members want her in a situation where she could become injured.

When asked how she felt a fall might influence her caregiver, CR001 stated, "I know he's very good at handling things. He's very strong, physically and mentally. So I really don't have a lot of worry about [CG001] and how he's reacting, is going to react if I fall.". When asked how she felt a fall would impact her caregiver and other family members, CR004 stated, "they would probably be relieved." CR004 described that the "relief" was relief that a fall would mean she would likely have to move out her home which would relieve her caregiver as there is a great deal of concern for her living alone in a relatively inaccessible home.

Caregiver Experiences

Two of the four caregivers in this investigation were spouses of the care recipient (CG001, CG003), one was the daughter of the care recipient (CG002) and the final caregiver was the daughter-in-law of the care recipient (CG004). Despite the relationship variation in the sample of caregivers they did have shared experiences regarding their concerns related to their care recipients falling. All four caregivers verbally reported that they had concerns about their care recipient falling, which was an inclusion criterion for this investigation. Upon completion of the three-interview process, the primary investigator understood the essence of the caregiver experience with respect of FoF to exist at the intersection of the biological, psychological, and social factors they experienced as a result of their caregiver fall concern. The intersection of these three factors manifested within the theme of the burden of caregiving with respect to fall concerns (Figure 5). Additional themes that supported the essence of the caregiver's experience with concern of the care recipient falling included: reasons for the caregiver fall concern, and compartmentalization during a fall emergency (Table 3).

Burden of Caregiving with Respect to Fall Concerns

Burden of caregiving with respect of falls concerns transcends all three aspects of the biopsychosocial model (Figure 5). The caregivers in this investigation discussed experiences with burden such as the added physical assistance they had to provide to both prevent a fall and/or assist following one; the disruption to their daily lives; the cognitive dissonance they experienced in their caregiving duties; and their experiences having to maintain their care recipient's autonomy in light of their concerns. The burden discussed by these caregivers with respect to their fall concerns was evidenced by their desires to manage the fall risk of the care recipient.

Managing the fall risk impacted the caregivers physically, in that they reported actively providing support or modifying the home environment of the care recipient to limit fall risk. They reported being impacted socially, when out with the care recipient because the caregiver must remain in a heighted state of awareness to not only keep themselves safe as a support but also be aware of additional threats to the stability of the care recipient. Additionally, the caregivers reported being impacted psychologically due to the increased stress and anxiety associated with their efforts in preventing falls CG001 said:

> It's always in the back of my mind, well, if something happens to her, you know. So that's why the way to deal with a lot of that risk is just for me to be there with her to minimize the amount of time that I'm not around.

The physical manifestations of the caregiver's concern of the care recipient falling includes modification to their own daily routine to maintain safety of the care recipient both in the home and out in the community. The caregivers in this study made conscious decisions to change their own behaviors with the care recipient to prevent a fall. Some ways that the caregivers noted their CFC was manifesting were to do things together with the care recipient, to install cameras that are motion activated (CG002), to limit the amount of time the care recipient spends walking when out in the community, and physically checking on the safety of the care recipient. CG004 stated, "But if it's a little bit of a walk, it's tricky…You know, I've always got to park in the handicapped spot with her or, or it's too far." The way that the physical actions taken by the caregivers to manage their CFC were based on the care needs of the care recipients. Similarly, CG003 stated:

If he's going to go someplace and get out the walker. The bigger walker that he likes to take with him. I take that out. I take him up and down with a golf cart if he has any appointments down at the village center for anything …It's hard. You know, it means more work for meCG002 discussed her experiences following her decision to put motion activated cameras in her mother's home so that she could remotely monitor for falls. She stated:

> There's just some nights where my stress levels are too high. And I just put my phone on vibrate, because I just can't can't take it on. And I have felt very guilty a couple of times because yeah, I've you know, tried to live a somewhat normal life and go out with friends or do something. You know, and if I went out late at night, I would have a couple of cocktails. I turned my phone off, I wanted to go to bed and I wouldn't get up and be able to drive over or whatever. And that's a couple times when she's fallen and she was on the ground for five hours. But of course, nobody else has an app for my camera or wants one or feels that they need that because I am the chosen one to be alerted since it was my idea. So yeah, it's a lot.

CG002 cited feelings of guilt and high levels of stress when she has attempted to distance herself from her caregiving duties.

The caregivers in this investigation reported a heightened awareness of their environment when they were out with the care recipient. That in turn caused them to take action to maintain the safety of the care recipient. CG001 stated, "It certainly gets me in a heightened sense of yeah, be careful yourself. Make sure you're stable. Adjust, adjust yourself so that you're a good solid support for her." CG001 went on to discuss how a local soccer facility caused him to be hyperaware of his surroundings to limit his wife's fall risk. He stated:

So, the soccer fields go within like a couple of feet at a wall. And at the end of the field, of course, is where the goal is. And the goal has nets. And the nets lay down on the on the ground, right at the back of the goal. And so when you're walking along, you got the space about yay big [holds up hands to less than two feet of space]. And the nets right there. If you're not careful, your foot goes in the net and catches your foot and down you go. And in fact, I was walking along, CR001 behind me using her cane. And I was thinking to myself, geez, you know, she catches her foot and goes down. So, I was looking at it.

The caregivers in this study responded to situations where their care recipient may be at an increased fall risk by expressing a hyper awareness of the surrounding environment. In the case of CG001 this meant increased physical support that was given to his care recipient.

Figure 5

Essence of Caregiver's Concern of the Care Recipient Falling

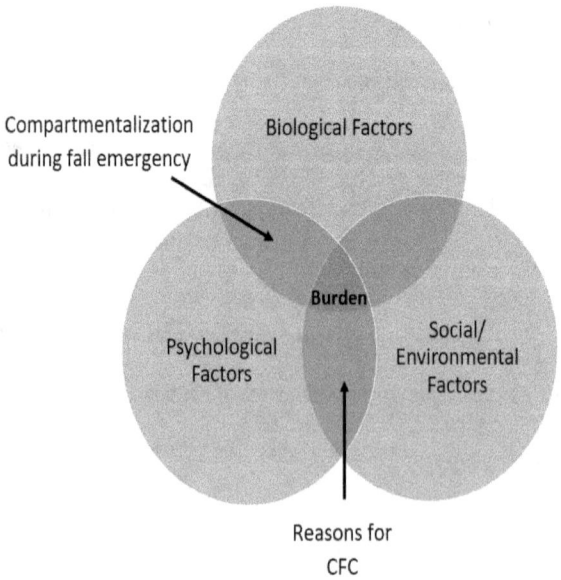

Reasons for Caregiver Fall Concern

All caregivers in this investigation reported they had concerns of the care recipient falling. The reasons behind the caregiver fall concern spanned the intersection of the psychological and social factors associated with the caregiver fall concern (Figure 5). These concerns were measured using the Caregiver Fall Concern Instrument (CFC-I). Scores ranged from 47/85 to 85/85. The reasons given for the concerns varied across the dyads. Some caregivers were concerned because of past history with falls, others were concerned because of the physical limitations of the care recipient either lending themselves to a fall or preventing the care recipient from assisting after a fall. Some caregivers expressed they were concerned because of their own limitations that would limit their ability to help in the event of a fall. The most cited reason for caregiver fall concern was due to the caregiver's perception of the care recipient's limitations and thus their increased fall risk.

Perception of Care Recipient Limitations. The caregivers in this investigation were asked to share their viewpoint on their care recipient's limitations and how they felt those contributed to their own concerns for the care recipient falling. The caregivers reported restrictions in mobility, surgical history, and the impact of inactivity as reasons why they were concerned about their care recipients falling. The following quotations indicate the specific physical limitations that the caregivers perceive their care recipients to have that influence their caregiver fall concern. CG001 stated:

> Because of the surgery that she had on her abdomen and then the hernia that occurred after that her abdomen is just very large, it's as if she's way overweight…And that just really restricts her range of motion in a lot of in a lot of

cases and it also tends to make it dangerous if she does lose her balance, you know that she's gonna go down. And that's what I'm always afraid of is if she gets down how am I going to get her back up?"

CG001 acknowledged that because of his on impairments and those of CR001 the two are unable to independently handle a fall which increased his concern. CG003 reported specific limitations that she perceives to occur as a result of a urinary tract infection. When CR003 has fallen or come close the cause of his functional decline has always been a urinary tract infection. CG003 reported, "it always seems to involve a real weakness on his part, and the urgency [to go to the bathroom]. And when those. When those two things arrive, I know." These caregivers reported their perceptions of the physical impairments that their care recipients had that contributed to their CFC. Weakness and impaired flexibility/mobility from surgeries were noted as hindrances to the ability of the care recipient to assist if they were to fall and needed to get up off of the ground. CG002 noted muscle atrophy due to inactivity as the reason why her mother's physical capabilities have declined. She stated, "So a lot of the problem is now that she has, you know, weakness, like muscles have atrophied a bit. So, between muscle weakness, and then the double knees being able, or not being able to kneel on them." CG002 identified the atrophied muscles as one of the primary reasons for her fall concern, she also reported her mother's physical inability to kneel which limits the ways in which she can get her mother off the ground in the event of a fall.

Traumatic Experiences with Falls. As each of the care recipients had fallen either prior to or during the course of this study, the caregivers described traumatic experiences associated with the falls that influenced their concerns for the care recipient falling again. Each of the caregivers who were with the care recipient as they fell described the traumatic nature of the fall in great detail. Others described the traumatic aftermath of the fall as they were not there to assist immediately following the fall event. CG001, in particular, had an added layer of trauma from the falls as his wife fell due to three separate medical emergencies that he believed to have been caused by a stroke. He stated:

> Well, they all come down to the same thing. And I'm scared to death that she's having a stroke. Because I've seen people with strokes. And I know how those that can drag on for years and years and years and years and years. You know, and it's horrible for the people that had the stroke. And it's horrible for the people that are the caregivers and it's not a not a pretty picture.

CG001 described three significant events that resulted in a CR001 falling all of which were true medical emergencies rather than her falling on her own due to some other impairment. For him the immediate concern is that a stroke has occurred due to her loss of consciousness during each fall.

Compartmentalization During a Fall Emergency

All four care recipients in this investigation had fallen such that the caregiver needed to become involved. This idea of compartmentalization during a fall emergency intersects the biological and psychological aspects of the biopsychosocial framework (Figure 5). The following four quotations are each caregivers' experiences immediately after seeing or hearing about their care recipient falling:

Well, I really wasn't thinking a whole lot, it was just more a matter of okay, let's, let's get, let's get the medics over here to, to get her to the hospital. And let's, let's immediately take care of whatever it is (CG001).

CG002 (referring to herself in the third person) goes into panic mode. And basically, medical mode. I mean, I, I literally just feel like, okay, I've got to treat her medically, possibly when I get there. Utilize whatever knowledge I have. You know, and you know, I am CPR certified again, and, and first aid and whatnot…So I feel like I, that's how I feel. I just feel like I'm I don't know, like, I'm on panic, because I'm nervous. But I also feel like this is my obligation. I have to hurry up and get there almost like an EMT or whatever. And assess the situation. And, you know, as long as she's okay, and she's not hit her head, you know, I tried to check her over. I do the best I can (CG002).

Shock. Just watching it happen. Just not any thought at all, except he's going down, he's going down. And as soon as he hit, I picked up the phone and called 911." "At the time, I was very cool and collected, luckily. But afterwards, after they took him to the hospital, I went back to pick up the chair and move things back around, and then I could see the blood all over, then it became like a major issue at that point (CG003).

Charles [pseudonym] and I were together, within the car, and we were like, Okay, what are we going to do? Let's get there first and we'll see what's happened. And if we got to go to the ER, we gotta go to the ER. And if we've gotta call an ambulance we call an ambulance. So let's get there first. We had Ren [pseudonym] on the phone too who was saying she's alright. She's in the chair.

I've got ice on her yeah, she's talking, you know, so. talked us through it (CG004).

Upon either seeing the fall or getting notified of the fall all the caregivers reported that they had to compartmentalize their emotions/concerns during the immediate aftermath of the fall with their first thought being to get the appropriate medical treatment. The feelings and thoughts that were associated with the meaning of the fall came later after the medical needs were tended to.

Dyad Experiences

The unique experiences of the dyads did not clearly fit into biological, psychological, and social/environmental considerations as the caregiver and care recipient experiences. That being said, the essence of fear of falling respective to the dyads was highlighted by themes that demonstrated how the dyads addressed concerns regarding the meaning of fall. Both the caregivers and care recipients described what it would mean to them if the care recipient were to fall. The care recipients described a general threat to their autonomy, where the caregivers discussed what it would mean in terms of increased physical assistance. Where the dyads differ from the individual experiences is how they make decisions to limit both the threat to autonomy as well as the increased needs that would be associated with a fall. The themes that emerged unique to the dyad experiences were: planning for the future and limiting burden.

The additional themes that emerged from the data analysis process spoke more to the nature of the relationship, and are better explained in the context of relational turbulence theory. The overarching theme is sources of relational turbulence, with the subthemes of communication regarding fall concerns and mismatch of perceptions regarding care recipient fall risk and physical limitations.

Planning for the Future

Both caregivers and care recipients expressed the idea that they were making decisions in preparation of potential future needs that could arise following a fall or some other medical emergency that might cause a decline in function. These plans were mutual decisions made by the caregivers and care recipients, with occasional outside influence from other family members and occasionally health care providers (Dyad002). The plans involve large scale home modifications or moving to places where higher levels of care are available if needed. CG001 stated:

> LeAnn [pseudonym] is looking at that now and saying you know, Dad, instead of having to go up and down stairs, it may get to a point sooner rather than later that you're going to want to put a bed down in that room. If not for one of you or both of you. And that bathroom just isn't geared up for it. And it's true the door is in the wrong position, etc. And so, in fact we were on the phone last night discussing that at length. How best to set that up to get it set up for when she needs to be down there. You don't want to wait till the last minute to have to have that done.

Both CG003 and CR003 discussed their move to a continuing care facility as a plan they made together in light of their increasing age and potential need for higher levels of care. CR003 stated:

> We were living in Georgia at the time … But that situation itself created a problem that we were isolated. We live probably 15 miles from the nearest hospital. [CG003's] sight began to decline due to macular degeneration. So, we

had then that or precipitated a concern that if anything did happen to me, transporting me to the hospital might be impossible, because she couldn't see she couldn't drive... And it made sense, because here we have this is what's called a continuing care community. We now live independently, there are a lot of services provided to us ... Then, if you need it, however, all right on site, there is skilled nursing. There is a memory unit. Hopefully I'll never get there. And an assisted living unit. So, there are three levels of deeper support that are available right here on campus. So, it gives you that a sense of you don't have to worry about that. You know, it's if it comes to and hopefully it won't, you know, it's here.

Despite the fact that they moved specifically to that location for the advanced care opportunities, in light of recent events, CG003 noted that it would likely be CR003 who resists needs the advanced care. She stated that, "... he'll be thinking of anything he can think of, to avoid going over there. And yet, that's the reason why we're here. You know, so that he can get care or I can, you know, depending on what happens ..."

The participants in this investigation spoke of the idea that while a physical change either to their home or into increased care would logistically be easy, there was still hesitation and reluctance to do so because of what those transitions indicate in terms of independence and autonomy.

Limiting Burden

The caregivers and care recipients included in this investigation both expressed a want to limit the burden either on their caregivers or on others who are involved in the lives of the dyads. Care recipients spoke of making decisions to spread out the burden or wanting to be more independent to limit their reliance on their caregivers.

Between interviews two and three, CR003 was hospitalized for an acute medical condition which resulted in significant decline in his ability to carry out his self-care activities independently due to the fact that he was unable to stand for any extended periods of time. When it came time for hospital discharge, CR003 stated that he advocated that he be discharged to a rehabilitation facility rather than home because, "I just didn't want to come home at that point and be a burden on [CG003]." Further discussion on this topic led CR003 to state:

> She would feel that she had more of a responsibility to be my 24/7 caregiver [more] than she already is. And I really don't want to put that burden on her. I want to be able to, again, handle any mobility issues on my own to avoid that fall but if I do fall, yeah, it's gonna be, it's gonna be a major change. I don't know what that change might entail. I have really no idea. But I just know it won't be good. It's likely to be bad.

CR003 indicted that despite his acknowledgement that he needs caregiver assistance that it would be an added burden for his caregiver to provide mobility and self-care assistance which he would like to avoid.

CG001, due to concern that he is unable to physically assist his wife from the group if she were to fall, expressed the idea of not wanting to call emergency services in the event of a fall resulting from a non-medical emergency. He reported that he went to his two neighbors who are younger and more physically able than himself and asked if they would be willing to be his first line of support in the event that CR001 fell. When asked how CG001 felt CR001 would respond that he said, "Well, I hope you don't have to. I'd hate for you to bother the neighbors. I'm glad you did that. But I hope you don't have to."

CR004 stated, "Well, I don't want to have to depend on everybody." She expressed not wanting to burden others to assist with her care. Given that her caregiving needs are the direct result of a fall she has been trying to improve her function so that she can drive herself and not rely on others. None of her family has stated that going to get her is problematic, however she feels that it is and does not want to rely on others for care.

Sources of Relational Turbulence

The participants in this investigation were asked to reflect if they felt their relationship with the other member of the dyad had changed at all based on the caregiving need around fall concerns. The responses were different, some individuals reporting "no" there was no change in the dynamic (Dyad001), while others reported that because of the nature of their relationship with the other member of the dyad that there was a change in their relational dynamic particularly with regards to the concern for falls. CG004 stated that she felt she became closer with her mother-in-law (CR004) because she fell into the caregiving role as she was newly retired and had the availability to care for CR004 after her fall. CG004 said:

> I actually think I talk to her more than her son and her daughter do. I think they don't ask her the questions or chat about things as much as I do. No, I think she talks with me much more than she talks to either one of them. So spending more time with me.

Dyad003 had a unique relationship where they married much later in life after previous relationships. For that reason, CG003 reported that she values their remaining time and wants CR003 to remain healthy and independent so they can enjoy their time together. CG003 also noted, that she did not believe their relationship dynamic had changed because:

> We have this pattern of whenever you do something physical that you don't want to have done. The other person will say to you, we'll just don't do that…So when he gets off balance, and feels, I'll say, where are you afraid of falling? And he'll say yes. And I'll just say, don't do that. You know, we just kind of make a joke out of it. More than anything else.

CR003 reported that he does not want CG003 to have the fear of him falling to be impactful in her life. He said:

> I don't want to have her have that fear. I don't want to have her have that burden. But I mean, that's something that she will have to deal with herself. I don't want it to happen. I don't want her to be that concerned. But I know her nature, she will be concerned.

While some of the relational dynamic changes were positive or non-existent, there were sources of turbulence described by the dyads regarding communication around fall concerns as well as mismatched perceptions regarding the care recipients fall risk and physical impairments.

Communication Regarding Fall Concerns. All caregivers included in this investigation reported having concern regarding their care recipient falling, and three of four care recipients (CR001, CR002, and CR003) answered "yes" when asked over the phone if they were fearful of falling. That being said, approximately 88% of the participants in this investigation have concerns related to falling, yet there was very little communication within the dyads regarding those concerns. Some reported they simply did not want to discuss the issue, or wanted to wait for someone else to bring it up. Others noted that communication on the matter did not need to be formal as there was a mutual understanding of the concerns. The following quotations describe the experiences of the dyads regarding their conversations about falling and FoF. Per the dyads, these conversations were often situational and not full sit-down conversations. CR001 stated, "I might have mentioned it once or twice. I'm sure I've mentioned the fact that you know, because of my unsteady condition I might fall unless I have a cane with me. Certainly outside." The caregiver from Dyad001 stated, "Well, it's just whenever the situation comes up, that it would be a topic to talk about, we talk about it."

Other participants echoed the idea that the discussion around falls is situational. CG003 reported, "We only talk about it if one of those incidences occurred where he's gotten off balance or afterwards as a memory of what's actually happened." CG002 has attempted to bring up the conversation with little acceptance from the care recipient:

> A very brief conversation, because she doesn't want to hear it. So, you know, even with the hearing aids in and turned up, she'll still go, what? I don't want to talk about that kind of thing. But she'll just sit there and kind of just nonchalant really not say much. So I'm never really quite sure I am getting through. But I do bring up the topic. Topics of her falling or, or slipping up out of bed or whatever losing her balance is what I try how I tried to put it.

The participants in this investigation noted there was often a formal lack of conversation regarding fall concerns. When asked why he feels conversations are not occurring CR003 simply stated, "Just because I don't want to talk about that with her." CR004 noted that she does not bring up the issue herself because she would rather have someone else bring it up. She said, "Well, I just always thought, you know, let them bring it up. I don't know." CR004 cited her lack of interest in having the conversation stems back to her not having concern for falling and knowing that a discussion about falls will likely lead to a discussion about her needing to move out of her house which she does not want to do.

Mismatch in Perception of Care Recipient Fall Risk and Physical Impairments. Some of the dyads included in this investigation revealed there was a mismatch in the fall risk and perception of limitations of the care recipient which has led to increased caregiver fall concern. In the case of Dyad002, the care recipient's ability to perceive and comprehend her limitations is limited by her cognitive state. CG002 stated:

> She'll say, it happened too fast. You know, I just couldn't get up fast enough. I couldn't get to the bathroom. You know, I mean, and that's why she feels embarrassed. She says, because she's like, nobody should have to come over and clean me up and do all this. She thinks she can do it by herself still. And it's very evident, she cannot.

CR002's cognitive state as perceived by CG002 is reported as a major contributing factor to the mismatch in perceived limitations which is causing more stress on the caregiver because the care recipient doesn't have the awareness to not do something that could result in a fall. She has no concept of why she had fallen. In Dyad004 there is also a mismatch in fall risk as well as the goals of each member of the dyad. CG004 states, "I don't think she should drive at all. But it's definitely a goal for her." In dyad 004 there is a mismatch of goals between the caregiver and care recipient particularly in regards to driving, which due to a neck mobility issue is the main reason CR004 needs care and that if CR004 could drive herself again then she would not have to ask people to do things for her.

The Essence of Fear of Falling

The overall purpose of this investigation was to identify the essence of FoF as experienced by the care recipients, caregivers, and dyads included in the study. In answering the three respective research questions, the essence of FoF and caregiver concern for falling were identified individually. However, there was as commonality across the experiences of care recipients, caregivers, and dyad experiences: preservation of way of life. For the care recipients preserving daily life means maintaining independence and limiting the threats to autonomy due to fall risk. For the caregivers, their efforts are aimed at maintaining the safety and stability of the care recipients so that they do not require higher levels of care, thus preserving the level of care being provided. For the dyads, preserving the way life manifested as making decisions that allow for supports to be in place as needs change in response to the aging process.

Chapter 5: Discussion

Literature surrounding the study of FoF has been successful in identifying risk factors of the development, developing scales to assess, and determining interventions to treat it (Bower et al., 2015; Delebaere et al., 2010a; de Souza et al., 2022; Hauer et al., 2010; Helbostad et al., 2010; Lavedán et al., 2018; Lee et al., 2018; Liu, 2015; MacKay et al., 2021; Öztürk et al., 2020; Tinetti et al., 1990; Tinetti & Powell, 1993; Vellas et al., 1997; Whipple et al., 2018; Yardley et al., 2005; Zijlstra et al., 2007). Risk factors that have been identified to be associated with the development of FoF fall into biological, psychological, and social/environmental considerations, which are discussed more in depth elsewhere in this paper. Increased social interaction is considered a protective factor against the development of FoF (Lee et al., 2018, MacKay et al., 2021). Current research, however, fails to identify if there is a point at which increased social interaction can actually increase fear of falling. An emerging body of literature has focused on caregiver concern of a care recipient falling (Ang et al., 2020b; Yang et al., 2019). Research efforts seeking to understand FoF and caregiver concern of the care recipient falling are largely confined to specific populations; either the caregivers or older adults. This investigation sought to recruit both caregivers and care recipients of the same caregiving dyad to assess their unique experiences regarding their fall concerns.

This investigation recruited caregivers who were over the age of 18, were providing unpaid care to a close friend or relative for at least one ADL or IADL, and expressed a verbal concern of their care recipient falling. Care recipients were included in this study if they were aged 65 or older, living freely in the community, and were able to communicate independently with the absence of severe cognitive impairment (MoCA score >10/30). The overall purpose of this investigation was to identify the essence of FoF as experienced by the care recipients, caregivers, and dyadic unit who were recruited into the study. Utilizing the phenomenological tradition, the principal investigator aimed to answer three distinct research questions utilizing the biopsychosocial model as a conceptual framework (Figure 3):

Research Question 1: How do older adults who receive care experience FoF in their daily lives considering biological, psychological, and social domains?

Research Question 2: How do caregivers of older adults experience fear of their care recipient falling considering biological, psychological, and social domains?

Research Question 3: How do caregiver - care recipient dyads uniquely experience FoF in daily life beyond individual experiences considering biological, psychological, and social domains?

Upon completion of the three step semi-structured interview process, the principal investigator identified not only the essence of FoF as it was experienced by the care recipients, caregivers, and dyads individually; but also came to understand the shared essence of FoF amongst this research sample. Regarding the experiences of the care recipients the following themes and subthemes emerged inductively from the literature: threats to autonomy, acceptance, maintenance of independence, and influence of the caregivers. Inductive themes that summarized the experiences of the caregivers included in this study were: burden of caregiving with respect to caregiver fall concern; reasons for caregiver fall concern, and compartmentalization during a fall emergency. The experiences that were unique to the dyad as a whole included the following themes and subthemes: planning for the future; limiting burden; communication regarding fall concern; and perception of the care recipient's physical limitations and fall risk. The shared essence across all subgroups of this study was the desire to preserve the way of life.

In identifying both the individual experiences and shared essence, the findings of this study can be implicated in the clinical interview process of older adults with fear of falling. In addition, the results also demonstrate the potential need for interprofessional management of individuals with fear of falling when there is the added dynamic of a caregiver. The remainder of this chapter includes an in-depth analysis of the results of this investigation, implications of the results of this study, and limitations of the study. This section concludes with overall conclusions.

Understanding the Essence of Fear of Falling

The purpose of this investigation was to identify the essence of FoF as described by the participants (caregivers, care recipients, and dyads) included in this study; which was identified as: preservation of way of life. Preserving the way of life encompasses the experiences of the caregivers, care recipients and dyads. The care recipients, who have become fearful of falling due to the threat a fall would pose to their autonomy, developed strategies to maintain their independence and thus their way of life. The caregivers described many ways in which they are attempting to preserve their way of life by managing the fall risk of their care recipients. By managing the care recipient fall risk, the caregivers can preserve the current status of their caregiving duties. The dyads are working together to make decisions that will allow them to preserve their way of life through modification to the home environment, and planning for a future decline in care recipient function.

Essence of Care Recipient Experiences

Research question one aimed to explore how older adults receiving care from an unpaid familial caregiver experience FoF under the consideration of biological, psychological and social/environmental domains. With the biopsychosocial model guiding the analysis process four inductive themes emerged from care recipient interviews: threats to autonomy, acceptance, maintenance of independence, and influence of the caregiver. These four themes speak to the essence of FoF as described by the care recipients included in this investigation (Figure 3). The theme "threats to autonomy" encompassed the intersection of the biological, psychological, and social factors that made up the care recipients experience with FoF. Acceptance, in terms of fall risk and self-awareness of physical limitations is situated at the intersection of the biological and psychological experiences of the care recipients with respect to FoF. The ability of the care recipients to utilize strategies to maintain their independence was identified to intersect the biological and social factors associated with fear of falling. Lastly, the influence of the caregiver was situated at the intersection of the psychological and social factors associated with care recipient FoF.

Given that all of the care recipients in this investigation were over the age of 65, their experiences regarding FoF can be discussed in terms of various theories of aging. As they currently stand, theories of aging fall into biological, social, and psychological theories (Mavritsakis et al., 2020). The biological theories of aging have much promise from intervention within the biomedical field, however they are outside the scope of what this investigation informs. Social and psychological theories of aging, however, are informed by the findings of this study.

Social Theories of Aging

Social theories of aging address how aging individuals interact with society as well as how their societal role changes throughout the aging process. Two opposing theories include activity theory and disengagement theory (Asiamah, 2017). Given the care recipients active participation in maintaining their independence, activity theory is an appropriate lens to examine the essence of fear of falling as experienced by the care recipients.

Activity theory hypothesizes that life satisfaction comes from higher levels of social interaction and activity (Knapp, 1977). The theory suggests that as individuals age, they should remain as socially active as they were in their middle-aged years (Knapp, 1977). Activity theory supports existing knowledge regarding the social context of FoF in individuals over age 65 (Auais et al., 2017, Lavedán et al., 2018; Lee et al., 2018; Liu, 2015; MacKay et al., 2021; Vellas et al., 1997). Less social interaction, discomfort with the neighborhood environment, and less access to community facilities were found to be associated with higher FoF in individuals over the age of 65 (Lee et al., 2018; MacKay et al., 2021). Through the techniques utilized by the care recipients to maintain their independence, use of assistive devices and modification of the home environment, they are able to stay active in their homes and communities in spite of their fear of falling.

Psychological Theories of Aging

Psychological theories of aging attempt to explain the aging process with respect to "mental processes, emotions, attitudes, motivation, and personality development" (Mavritsakis et al., 2020, p. 255). An additional consideration for exploring the essence of FoF relative to care recipient experiences is the selection, optimization, and compensation (SOC) theory. SOC theory suggests that older adults do not passively accept loss, but instead they cope with losses with selection of new life goals, optimizing their available resources to meet those goals, and using compensatory strategies to work towards their goals (Baltes, 1997; Gondo et al., 2013). The theme of acceptance is explored in light of the SOC theory. The care recipients in this investigation expressed an acceptance of their declining physical status and therefore increased fall risk. In light of that, none expressed activity avoidance due to their concerns which suggests they are strategizing ways to navigate their lives being respectful of the self-identified physical limitations, and making new goals to remain safe while continuing to do their desired activities. These processes fall in line with the SOC theory.

Developmental Theories. Developmental theories are largely utilized to understand childhood, adolescent, and young adult development (Elder, 1998; Maree, 2021). Erikson's psychosocial development theory has been well studied in children and adolescents (Maree, 2021). The theme of threats to the care recipient autonomy can be discussed in terms of Erikson's stage eight: ego integrity versus despair. Ego integrity is experienced when an older adult, "accepts his or her life cycle as something that had to be, feels connected to others, and experiences a sense of wholeness, meaning and coherence as he or she faces (the approach of) death" (Kleijn et al., 2016, p. 2). Despair, was identified as the older adult experiencing, "regret about the life he or she has led, and has feelings of sadness, failure, and hopelessness" (Kleijn et al., 2016, p. 2). When asked, "what would falling mean to you?", the care recipients described not only physical ramifications but also threats to their autonomy. As falling would pose a threat to the autonomy of the care recipients, that threat could hinder the experience of ego- integrity. The care recipients exercise increased caution in their daily activities to avoid a fall, and the potential for the despair that comes with it. By exercising caution and being concerned about falling, these care recipients are putting themselves in a position to achieve ego integrity.

Influence of the Caregiver

Due to the nature of this study, there were influences coming from the caregivers that impacted the care recipient experiences with FoF. These influences fall outside the scope of the psychological and social theories of aging discussed above, however they still have merit in terms of contributing to the essence of the care recipient FoF. As stated elsewhere, increased social support was cited as a protective factor against the development of FoF (Lee et al., 2018; MacKay et al., 2021). However, the literature surrounding fear of falling has yet to identify if there is a point at which increased social support can actually be a risk factor for the development of FoF. Two care recipients noted that their caregivers were justified in their concern due to witnessing a past fall and observing their mobility deficits. The care recipients expressed that they appreciated the willingness of the caregiver to aid in their safety to prevent falls and make sure they stay on top of emerging health concerns. The care recipients were asked how they felt a fall would impact their caregivers. One care recipient expressed that nothing would really change because mentally and physically she felt her caregiver could manage any issues that may arise. Another care recipient felt that if she fell again, it would mean that her caregiver and other family members would make her move out of her home to a more accessible location given her age and mobility deficits. That particular care recipient did not express that she herself was fearful of falling due to her activity level with an emphasis on maintaining her leg strength and balance. Despite the fact that she believed falling would mean she has to move because of her caregiver's wants, it was not enough to cause her to experience FoF. Based on the results of this investigation, the care recipients did not express a negative influence coming from the caregivers. Future exploration could investigate this idea further.

Essence of Caregiver Experiences

The second research question for this investigation aimed to explore the essence of the caregiver's experience of caregiver concern of the care recipient falling within the context of the biopsychosocial model. At the intersection of the biological, psychological, and social factors associated with the caregiver experience was the theme: burden of caregiving with respect to caregiver fall concerns. Additional themes that contributed to the essence of the caregiver experience included reasons for caregiver fall concern, and compartmentalization during a fall emergency. Reasons for caregiver fall concern is situated at the intersection of the psychological and social factors associated with the caregiver fall concern. The theme "compartmentalization during a fall emergency" takes into account the biological and psychological experiences of the caregivers.

Caregiving literature in large part focuses on the negative outcomes and burden associated with caregiving. The CDC (2022b) identified that individuals who provide informal care are at risk for higher levels of depression and anxiety, worsened immune function, poorer self-reported health, increased mental health concerns, and higher instances of premature death. The experiences described by the caregivers in this investigation focused more on the burden associated with caregiving in light of their fall concerns rather than any satisfaction they felt in providing safety and stability to the care recipients who were likewise concerned about falling.

Burden of Caregiving with Respect to Fall Concerns

The theme of "burden of caregiving with respect to fall concerns" best highlights the multifactorial nature of the caregivers' experiences regarding their concern of their care recipient falling. Physically speaking, these caregivers were active in providing support to their care recipients to aid in the prevention of a fall, which in one case resulted in lower back discomfort for the caregiver. Three of four care recipients had experienced a significant fall within this last year and one fell three times during the course of data collection for this investigation. These caregivers are also involved in providing the physical assistance to get the participant up following a fall. One caregiver expressed that one of his major concerns is the fact that he cannot physically get his care recipient off the ground if she were to fall and that he had to call 9-1-1 to assist him in the past. Ang et al. (2019a) cited that caregiver fall concern was influenced by a number of factors related to the behaviors and perceptions of the caregiver and care recipient in addition to the ways in which the caregiver attempted to manage the fall risk of the care recipient. By providing physical assistance to prevent a fall, the caregivers were actually able to control some of the fall risk and potentially decrease some of their concern. The outcome of a previous fall was also acknowledged as a factor contributing to caregiver fall concern (Ang et al., 2020b). For the caregivers in this investigation, some falls resulted in trips to the emergency room and a greater need for care. These fall outcomes contribute to perpetuating the fall concern of the caregivers.

The caregivers in this investigation expressed a mismatch in their internal feelings and outward actions regarding the care they were providing regarding their fall concerns. This idea was interpreted as cognitive dissonance with the caregiving responsibilities. Cognitive dissonance is described as the resulting mismatch between what one believes they should think or feel and how they actually think or feel (Elliot & Devine, 1994; Festinger & Carlsmith, 1959). The caregivers noted that despite frustration in having to provide care and assistance to limit the probability of the care recipient falling they did so with compassion. One caregiver described in an attempt to limit his outward frustrations he and his care recipient have altered their nightly routine to lessen the effects of fatigue. The disruption of daily life produced by the caregiver's concerns is another contributing factor to the burden described by the caregivers in this investigation. This disruption is also likely contributing towards the feelings of cognitive dissonance for the caregivers in this investigation. They are contending with a loss of their own independence for fear that something will happen to the care recipient if they are not with them, and yet still have to provide the assistance needed to prevent a fall.

The caregivers also expressed struggles with maintaining the autonomy of their care recipients. Two of the four care recipients required care only for physical tasks. The additional two care recipients had evidence of mild and moderate cognitive impairment and required more assistance from the caregiver. The caregivers of the two care recipients who needed physical assistance only described this challenge with maintaining autonomy in light of their concerns. Ang et al. (2019a) identified that a source of caregiver fall concern was the care recipient's attitudes and behaviors around their own fall risk. The care recipients needing only physical assistance were well aware of their limitations which is why they were accepting care for them. In theory, the care recipients' acceptance of their limitations should alleviate the caregiver concern, however, it did not.

The caregivers in this investigation expressed a heightened situational awareness when assisting the care recipient for fall related concerns. In addition, they noted changes they had made to the home and living environment of the care recipient to maintain their safety. By being more aware of the surrounding environment and knowing they have tried to modify the care recipients living environment to make it safer the caregivers are attempting to manage the fall risk of their care recipient. This finding is consistent with the work of Ang and colleagues (2019a). The authors identified that the care recipient living environment was a source of caregiver fall concern. As evidenced by the scores on the CFC-I (Table 2), the risk management techniques utilized by the caregivers have not yet alleviated their concerns.

Reasons for Caregiver Fall Concern

Ang et al. (2019a, 2020b) identified that caregiver fall concern is heightened by the outcome of a prior fall, lack of care recipient acceptance and awareness of their fall risk, propensity of the care recipient to ignore the caregiver attempts to manage their fall risk, the care recipients living environment, and the caregiver's perception of the care recipient overall health and fall risk. The results of this investigation highlighted that these caregivers all experienced a traumatic fall with their care recipients. Three caregivers noted that the fall resulted in either a trip to the emergency department or urgent care. During those traumatic falls the caregivers all described a process during which they compartmentalized during the immediate emergency. This indicates that there was a brief period of time where the caregiver's concern was second to the immediate medical need of their care recipient.

The caregivers were asked to describe what they perceived to be the factors contributing to the fall risk of their care recipients. Consistent with Ang et al. (2019a) the perceived health concerns and strength and mobility deficits were contributing factors to the caregivers' fall concerns.

Essence of Dyad Experiences

The third research question sought to identify the essence of the dyad's unique experience regarding FoF within the context of the biopsychosocial model. The dyadic experiences highlighted themes that impacted both the caregiver and care recipient. Upon completion of the analysis process, it appears that the goals of the dyad are to make decisions that allow both the caregiver and care recipient to continue to maintain their current balance in giving and receiving care in regards to FoF. The essence as identified in the dyad experiences included planning for the future and limiting burden. These two themes did not fall cleanly into the biopsychosocial framework. This is likely due to the fact that these themes incorporate the point of view of both the caregiver and the care recipient and for that reason what may be considered a biological factor for one may be a psychological or social factor for another. There were additional themes that emerged around the dyad experience regarding FoF, however they are better understood in the context of relational turbulence theory.

Planning for the Future

Both the caregivers and care recipients engaged in behaviors to manage the fall risk of the care recipient. Two of these dyads were spousal dyads meaning the caregiver was also of increasing age and experiencing mobility deficits. There is a possibility that the plans made on behalf of the care recipients could also benefit the caregivers in the future. For the other two dyads which consisted of a mother and daughter, and a mother-in-law and daughter-in-law, the planning for the future appeared to be aimed at keeping the care recipient safe in their home and not increasing the caregiving need due to a fall. In some cases, the caregivers felt that the care recipients were or would be resistive to the plans. The care recipients are actively engaged in processes to manage their own fall risk and thus maintain their independence. The thought that planning for the future means a change to the living environment or care plan can be attributed as another perceived threat to the autonomy of the care recipient.

Limiting Burden

As described by the dyads, limiting burden encompassed both the care recipient trying to limit the burden on their caregiver and the caregiver trying to limit burden on other individuals outside of the immediate dyad. Two care recipients expressed that they tried to handle situations themselves so that they did not increase the burden on their caregivers. One care recipient chose to go to a rehabilitation facility prior to being discharged home after a brief hospitalization because he did not want his caregiver to have to take on more than she is already doing. Another care recipient stated that she wanted to get better so she could drive again because she felt like a burden having to have people take care of her. When asked, the care recipient stated that her caregiver never said driving to her home was problematic. Perhaps in the case of these two care recipients, they are picking up on the cognitive dissonance experienced by the caregivers and trying to remain as independent as possible within the confines of their physical impairments.

One caregiver expressed that because he is physically unable to assist his care recipient if she were to fall, he would have no choice but to call emergency services even if there was not a pressing emergency need, which he did not want to do because that would burden the system. Instead, he chose to ask his neighbors if they would be ok with being the first line of assistance if there was not an actual medical emergency that caused the fall. He stated that when he told his care recipient of his plans, she expressed that she was happy he did it but that she did not want to bother the neighbors. Both members of this dyad expressed they did not want to burden others regarding their fall concerns.

Relational Considerations for Fear of Falling

Relational turbulence theory was identified as another theoretical lens for this investigation. Initially explored in the context of romantic relationships (Solomon & Knobloch, 2004; Solomon et al., 2016), relational turbulence theory posits that transitions in relationships are crucial time periods where uncertainty around relational roles resulting from the transitions can complicate the relationships as sources of turbulence, which in turn can positively or negatively influence the relationship .Relational turbulence theory is now being applied in the context of caregiving relationships (Knobloch et al., 2020). In the context of caregiving dynamics, the theory suggests that changes in level of independence cause transitions between caregivers and care recipients and the uncertainty associated with the transitions create turbulence with the caregiving relationship (Knobloch et al., 2020). Cooper and Pitts (2022) explored relational turbulence theory in caregiving dyads where the care recipient had either Alzheimer's Disease or other associated dementia. The authors found that in the absence of memory deficits most transitions into care have a settling in period where both the caregiver and care recipient adapt to their new roles; however, in the presence of significant memory impairment the dyads are in a more constant state of transition.

Within this sample, there were three different types of caregiving dyads: spousal dyads, one mother daughter dyad, and one mother-in-law/daughter-in-law dyad. Given the various types of caregiving dyads, there are special considerations in terms of how FoF is experienced. In the spousal dyads included in this investigation both members of the dyads were in their 80's. Both the caregivers and care recipients in these dyads had concerns regarding falls and general mobility and strength deficits. These differed from the parent-child and mother-in-law/daughter-in-law dyads where the caregivers were middle aged and did not worry about their own deficits, so all the focus was on the needs and risks of the care recipient. Two of the dyads reported that not much had changed in terms of the nature of the relationship in light of the care being provided for fall related concerns. One caregiver reported that she felt it improved the relationship with the care recipient because they have been able to spend more time with each other. Additionally, she felt that because of the increased time spent together she was able to communicate more with the care recipient than she had previously been able to. Despite the fact that these dyads did not report increased turbulence due to the transition into care they did cite some experiences that could be considered sources of turbulence. The first being communication regarding fall concerns, and the second being a mismatch in perceived fall risk of the care recipients.

During the final interview both members of the dyad were asked about their communication with the other person regarding fall concerns. One caregiver noted that during the times she has tried to bring it up, the care recipient pretends she cannot hear and does not engage in the conversation. A care recipient stated that she chooses not to bring it up for concern that her caregiver and other family members will want her to move to a more accessible location with one floor living. Other caregivers reported that when they do have discussions about falling or the concerns associated with it, the conversations are often situational where there has been a brief loss of balance or heightened concern that a fall will occur. In the cases where the care recipient is resistant to communication regarding falls, there is likely increased concerns from the caregiver because they may perceive that the care recipient is not taking their fall risk seriously. This is consistent with the findings of Ang et al. (2019a) who found that caregiver fall concern was influenced by care recipient attitudes about their own fall risk. Coincidentally, the score of the caregiver, whose care recipient would not participate in conversations about fall concerns, had the maximum possible score on the CFC-I (85/85).

Care recipients were asked to self-assess their limitations that may increase fall risk and/or FoF. Caregivers were asked to discuss their perceptions of the care recipients' limitations that increased fall risk and thus increased their concern for falls. In two dyads, the caregivers and care recipients shared the same perceptions of the care recipients' risk. However, in the other two dyads, there was a mismatch between caregiver perception and care recipient perception. This mismatch is another potential source of turbulence within the dyads. Ang and colleagues (2019a) also found that caregiver's perception of fall risk was associated with their concern for falls. In the cases where there was a mismatch in perceptions the caregivers self-reported higher levels of caregiver fall concern on the CFC-I. The care recipient of one dyad that had a mismatch in the perception of risk, also was found to moderate cognitive impairment according to her MoCA score (15/30). During the interview process, it became clear that the care recipient was not able to self-assess her physical impairments due to her cognitive impairment. She regularly stated that she thought she was "doing pretty good" given her age, she was unable to recall the fact that she had fallen three times between her first contact with the principal investigator and her interview. The caregiver of this care recipient was extremely concerned about falls (CFC-I score 85/85), which has caused a significant disruption to her daily life as a caregiver. The second dyad with a mismatch in perceptions of care recipient fall risk and physical limitations was not contending with the added concern of cognitive impairment. In both cases, the mismatch in perceptions was characterized by increased turbulence in the dyads. In the case of Dyad002, the findings of Cooper and Pitts (2022) can be applied given the cognitive status of CR002. Perhaps due to her memory impairments the dyad has not been able to settle into a consistent routine of care provided and care received, which could be responsible for the high levels of caregiver fall concern experienced by CG002.

Implications

The findings from this investigation have the potential to inform the clinical interview process for physical therapists treating older adults with FoF. The results of this study suggest that when a caregiver is involved with an older adult and they themselves have concerns about the older adult falling, a complex relational dynamic emerges that will need to be addressed. For this reason, the results of this investigation also have implications for interdisciplinary practice.

Clinical Implications for Physical Therapists

Physical therapy practice is guided in large part by the International Classification of Functioning, Disability and Health (ICF) framework, which indicates that a health condition is influenced by the body structures and their functions (or dysfunction), activities, participation, environmental factors, and personal factors (WHO, 2001 as cited by McDougal et al., 2010). This framework is similar to the biopsychosocial framework (Engel, 1977; Mosey, 1974) utilized to guide this inquiry, which allows parallels to be drawn from the results of this study to physical therapy practice. When a patient comes to physical therapy, they undergo an examination during which time the physical therapist takes a detailed history through a clinical interview and performs tests and measures to eventually make a diagnosis. The findings from this investigation hold particular importance for the clinical interview portion of examination. Physical therapists should be asking questions of their patients with fall related concerns how they perceive their own fall risk.

Delbaere and colleagues (2010b) investigated perceived versus actual physiological fall risk in a sample of older adults aged 70-90. The findings of this investigation are interesting in light of the various cognitive capacities of the care recipients included in this investigation. The authors identified four possible classifications based on the level of agreement between the perceived and physiological fall risk (Delbaere et al., 2010b). Individuals with low perceived fall risk and low physiological fall risk were identified as "vigorous", those with high perceived risk and low physiological risk were identified as "anxious", those with low perceive risk and high physiologic risk were identified as "stoic" and those with high physiological risk and high perceived risk were labeled "aware" (p. 4). When a physical therapist asks the patient to perceive their own fall risk, they can then perform the appropriate tests and measures to assess the physiological fall risk to see if there is agreement (Vigorous, Aware). All care recipients in this investigation acknowledged they were at risk for falls either due to their age or specific impairments of strength, mobility, and balance which is indicative of higher physiological fall risk, they also expressed that they were concerned about falling, and their FES-I scores showed their concern was valid. Physical therapists can utilize the FES-I along with a comprehensive fall risk assessment to determine the perceived and physiological risk for falls of their patients.

Additional considerations for physical therapy practice include the involvement of the caregiver. Three of four caregivers in this investigation managed the transportation needs of their care recipients and also accompanied them to doctor visits. When a caregiver is present at the examination, it is important for the therapist to remember to balance the concerns of the actual patient as well as giving time for the care recipients to share information. Additionally, past caregiving literature identified that unpaid or informal caregivers take on a significant role in terms of care delivery without proper training to safely deliver the care (Benton & Meyer, 2019; Jeyatheron et al., 2020; Lingler et al., 2008). Depending on the care need, informal or untrained caregivers are at an increased risk of sustaining musculoskeletal injuries themselves (Benton & Meyer, 2019). In the case of the caregivers in this investigation there was no formal training to assist their care recipients with fall concerns. This is likely because there was no single event that caused the caregiving to start, it was more in response to a general physical decline of the care recipient resulting in increased fall risk. Physical therapists can incorporate caregiver training into their plan of care determined at the initial examination. The caregiver training can address how to safely provide assistance to limit a fall as well as address strategies for both the caregiver and care recipient should a fall occur.

Implications for Interprofessional Collaboration

Physical therapists are well trained to evaluate and treat the biological processes that would contribute to FoF. Through cognitive-behavioral interventions, physical therapists are actually able to address some of the psychological and social/environmental factors that have been shown to contribute to FoF. Despite this, physical therapists cite they are uncomfortable with addressing the psychosocial considerations of disease due to inadequate training (Dalusio-King & Hebron, 2022). In the cases where physical therapists are unable to adequately address the psychological and social factors associated with FoF, it may be appropriate to seek additional treatment with a social work provider and/or a gerontologist. This investigation revealed there were individual and dyadic factors that influence the experiences with FoF. Navigating complex relationships is out of the scope of the physical therapists. In these instances, having the ability to refer to providers who can is paramount to prevent the FoF from getting worse.

Limitations

The biopsychosocial model (Engel 1977; Mosey, 1974) was the guiding framework for this investigation which utilized descriptive and essential phenomenological principles to investigate the essence of the caregiver -care recipient dyad respective to fear of falling. The theory and methods of choice have some inherent limitations for the interpretation of the results and analysis of this investigation.

Theoretical Limitations

The biopsychosocial model was proposed as a means to explore disease expression in the context of biological, psychological and social constructs (Engel, 1977; Mosey, 1974). The biopsychosocial model was chosen as the framework to guide this study, because FoF is often discussed in terms of biological, psychological, and social/environmental risk factors (Lavedan et al., 2018; Lee et al., 2018; Liu, 2015; MacKay et al., 2021; Ozturk et al., 2020; Vellas et al., 1997). A special consideration for social risk factors comes from the presence of a caregiver who may impact the functional independence of their care recipient due to their own concerns of the care recipient falling (Ang et al., 2019a; Yang, 2019; Yang et al., 2020). While the biopsychosocial model is an appropriate way to investigate the essence of the caregiver - care recipient dyad, it does limit the analysis of this investigation.

Methodological Limitations

The chosen methodology has historically been questioned regarding the rigor and applicability of findings to more general populations (Hallett, 1995; Priest, 2002). These limits were further compounded by the use of non-random sampling techniques (Taherdoost, 2016). By utilizing purposive sampling to identify participants that meet designated caregiver and care recipient criteria, the reach of the findings are limited from being transferable to the caregiver - care recipient dyad outside the context of FoF. This limit of transferability limits the rigor of the proposed study (Lincoln & Guba, 1985).

Staying true to the phenomenological tradition, this investigation had a small sample size, which allowed for more in-depth descriptions of the experiences with FoF. While a small sample size is acceptable given the methodology of choice, there were mixed types of dyads within the sample which limits the transferability of the findings. Further limiting transferability, and to some extent dependability, was the use of semi-structured interviews (Queirós et al., 2017). While an interview guide was utilized to identify questions that will be asked of all participants, the ability of the interview to be flexible and probing of ideas that emerge limit the ability of all of the questions to be reproduced. The use of a three-interview process was to enable the principal investigator to engage in iterative processes between interviews as each subsequent interview guide was developed. However, due to the cognitive limitations of one participant, one interview was conducted that encompassed all three interview guides. This allowed for the participant to complete the study, however limited the researcher from adapting between guides. The interviews were also supposed to be scheduled three to seven days following the previous interviews. All interview twos were scheduled within that time frame, however due to participant illness, some interview threes were conducted outside the seven-day timeframe that Seidman (2013) described.

The principal investigator utilized interpretive phenomenological analysis (IPA) rather than a traditional thematic analysis (Braun & Clarke, 2006; Colaizzi, 1973; Smith & Osborn, 2003). According to Braun and Clarke (2006), the themes from IPA are determined a priori from the guiding framework, where in a traditional thematic analysis the themes are found inductively in the data. In this investigation, biological, psychological and social themes were determined a priori. However, within those constructs, the themes were determined by the data itself. By limiting the nature of the themes into a biopsychosocial framework there is a chance that the chosen analysis missed additional themes that do not fit the framework.

An additional consideration for methodological limitations lies in the usage of the FES-I as the measure of care recipient FoF. A secondary finding of the systemic review conducted by MacKay and colleagues (2021) was the vast differences in the way in which fear of falling was measured. Of the 46 included studies, 29 used a single question to assess if a participant had fear of falling, 15 utilized at least one version of the Falls Efficacy Scale (FES), and additional scales (e.g., Activities Balance Confidence [ABC] Scale, Outdoor Fall Questionnaire, Fear Avoidance Behavior Questionnaire) were used much less frequently. The differences in measurement of fear of falling echo critiques of McKee (2002) and Liu (2015) who report difficulty in the ability to compare results of studies due to a lack of measurement standardization.

The different ways of measuring and operationalizing FoF call reported prevalence estimates into question. Studies where a single yes/no question was used to assess for fear of falling report significantly higher prevalence rates (Lee et al., 2018; Ozturk et al., 2020; Vellas et al., 1997). The Falls Efficacy Scale (FES), FES- I, or translated version of the FES are widely used (Liu, 2015; MacKay et al., 2021). The FES was established by Tinetti et al. (1990) and the international version was validated in 2005 (Yardley et al., 2005). Since that time, cutoff scores have been established (Delbaere et al., 2010a) and various versions to meet the needs of different international populations have been validated (Hauer et al., 2010; Helbostad et al., 2010). Despite the wide use of the FES, some have questioned its utility. McKee (2002) sought to determine if falls efficacy was able to independently measure fear of falling or if scores on the FES were more related to the ability of an individual to perform the ADL in question on the scale. The FES was found to address the ability of the individual to perform ADLs rather than measuring self-efficacy for limiting falls while performing the activity (McKee, 2002). When compared to a single question (yes/no), there was no association between scores on the FES and if that same person responded to the question as "yes", indicating they were fearful of falling (McKee, 2002). Solving the decades old issue regarding the measurement of FoF was beyond the scope of this study.

One final methodological limitation was that the interviews took place during the winter months in Upstate New York. The psychological impact of the weather at the time of the data collections could have impacted concerns about falling for both the caregivers and care recipients included in this investigation.

Bias

The principal investigator made efforts to reduce bias throughout the data collection and analysis process. By utilizing a co-coder to develop the initial codebook, and having the secondary codes validated with expert opinion. In spite of those efforts, there is still some inherent bias which poses a limitation to this investigation. As the principal investigator, co-coder, and the individual providing expert opinion are licensed physical therapists, there was a preference for the care recipient experience over that of the caregiver, as the care recipient would likely be the member of the dyad receiving physical therapy care. Additionally, due to the formal training of the principal investigator the implications for physical therapy and interdisciplinary practice were identified in the context of outpatient providers. The principal investigator aimed to mitigate the bias in data analysis by drawing on input from individuals in the social work field with training in gerontology. Qualitative research is gaining traction in healthcare research, however there are some ethical considerations to bear in mind when the professional training of the researcher creates a power differential with the participants. To combat this, the principal investigator acknowledged her licensure as a physical therapist at the start of the interview process, but made it clear that no professional advice would be given during the interview process. Participants were provided with a list of resources regarding concerns (Appendix L).

Suggestions for Future Work

This investigation utilized a phenomenological approach to investigate the essence of FoF amongst a sample of caregiving dyads where at least one member of that dyad expressed concern of the care recipient falling. The sample size was relatively small and within that there were a mix of dyad types. Future investigations would do well to find one uniform type of dyad to interview such as only spousal dyads or parent-child dyads. This investigation did not suggest that there was a point at which the caregiver fall concern became a risk factor for the care recipient's experiences with FoF. Additional research efforts could include analysis of the moderating effect of caregiver fall concern on measures of the care recipient FoF. Given the inconsistency in literature surrounding FoF on how to measure it, further research is needed to establish a uniform measure of FoF versus low falls efficacy, which will make comparisons in the literature more meaningful.

The principal investigator identified the shared essence of FoF amongst the study participants to be "preservation of way of life". A model theorizing this idea is proposed in Figure 6. Future investigations could evaluate this model in the context of caregiving dyads where FoF and/or caregiver fall concern are present.

Figure 6

Shared Essence of Fear of Falling

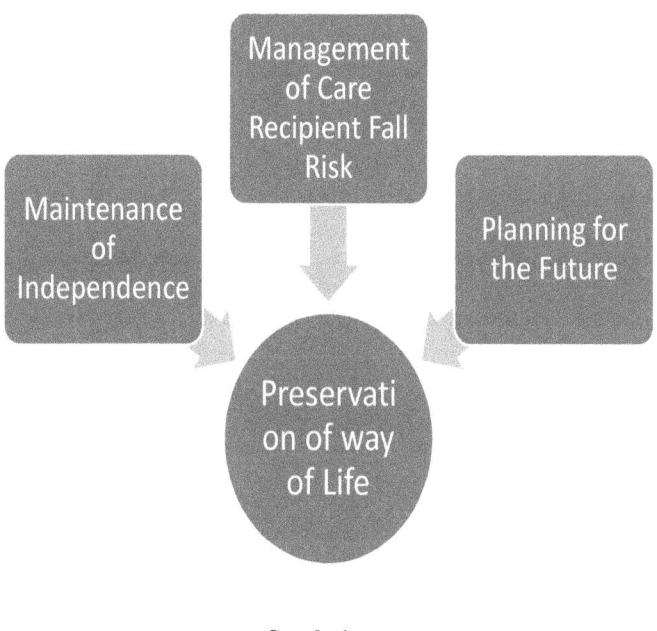

Conclusions

This investigation aimed to identify the essence of FoF as it was experienced in the context of caregiving dyads through a biopsychosocial lens. The individual experiences of the caregivers and care recipients recruited into this study were able to be captured by the biopsychosocial model. The care recipient's experiences encompassed the themes of: threats to autonomy, acceptance of fall risk, maintenance of independence, and influence of the caregiver. Caregiver experiences included the following themes:

burden with respect to fall concerns, reasons for caregiver fall concern, and compartmentalization during a fall emergency. Dyad experiences with respect for fear of falling included planning for the future and limiting burden. The experiences of dyads however were better understood through relational turbulence theory. The shared common essence of FoF as identified in this investigation was the need to preserve the way of life. The findings of this investigation have implications for the physical therapy evaluation process for older adults with FoF and who may have a caregiver assisting them in their daily lives. Due to the complex interaction of psychological and social factors contributing to FoF, as well as the relational dynamic between the caregiver and care recipient, physical therapists may need to refer their patients with FoF to providers who are able to address all of those additional influences. The principal investigator looks forward to further exploration of the concepts identified in this investigation.

www.ingramcontent.com/pod-product-compliance
Lightning Source LLC
LaVergne TN
LVHW011949070526
838202LV00054B/4867